HIVES

The Road To Diagnosis and Treatment of Urticaria

A Workbook and Resource

for Healthcare Professionals and Patients

ENCOURAGES A COOPERATIVE APPROACH BETWEEN

HEALTHCARE PROFESSIONALS AND PATIENTS THAT IMPROVES OUTCOMES

A TIME-SAVING METHOD THAT ORGANIZES AND STANDARDIZES

THE EVALUATION AND TREATMENT

ALAN A. WANDERER, M.D.

AnsonPublishing, LLC

Bozeman, Montana

AnsonPublishing, LLC

Copy Editors: Patricia Wanderer and Janet Stewart
Layout Editor: Dianne Nelson, Shadow Canyon Graphics, Golden, Colorado
    E-mail: dnshadow@earthlink.net
Cover Design: Lisa Rickenbaugh, Collage Graphic Design, Bozeman, Montana

First Edition 2004
10 9 8 7 6 5 4 3 2 1

Copyright© by AnsonPublishing, LLC.

Printed in the United States of America

AnsonPublishing, LLC
2055 North 22nd Ave.
Suite 1
Bozeman, MT 59718
USA
Tel: 1-866-307-1112
E-mail: ansonpublishing@aacpc.com
Web site: www.aacr.salu.net
       www.alanwanderermd.com
International Standard Book Number: 0-9727948-0-8

Library of Congress Control Number: 2003092024
Hives (Urticaria) / Swelling (Angioedema) / diagnosis / treatment

Readers are advised to check the current product information/insert provided by the manufacturer for each drug and/or medical device to verify recommended dosage, method and duration of administration, drug-drug interactions, warnings and contraindications. It is the responsibility of the healthcare provider to determine FDA status of a drug or device for use in clinical practice. Despite extreme care to confirm the accuracy of the presented information, the author, editor and publisher are not responsible for errors or omissions and make no warranty, expressed or implied, with regard to the currency, completeness or accuracy of the contents of this publication. The author, editor and publisher disclaim all liability occurring directly or indirectly from the use or application of any information contained in this book. The information contained in this book is not intended to replace the advice of a healthcare professional. Patients are advised and encouraged to consult a healthcare professional regarding the diagnosis and treatment of their health condition.

Acknowledgments

Special appreciation to Beth and Bill Sagstetter, two accomplished people who encouraged and guided me through the maze of authoring and publishing this book.

A particular thanks to the following who provided academic assistance and constructive critique during the writing of this book: David Goodman M.D.; Patricia Giclas Ph.D.; David Pearlman M.D; Hal Hoffman M.D.; Richard Asarch M.D.; and especially Charles Kirkpatrick M.D. for his supportive comments in the foreword.

I would also like to mention individuals who have been inspirational role models in my life and career. They are: Richard Farr M.D. (In memoriam); Hyman Chai M.D. (In memoriam); David Starrett M.D.; Henry Shinefield M.D., Lawrence Strong Ph.D. and Elliot Ellis, M.D.

A special thanks to special friends who have been there when I needed them: Edwin Bronsky M.D.; John Winder M.D.; Carol and Larry Laycob M.D.; and Elaine and Richard Asarch M.D.

For

My *brothers Richard, Warren, Paul, and Bob;*

My *children Rob and Wendy, Kristin and Steve, David and Dani, and Jennifer;*

My *grandchildren Mitchell, Duncan, Rian, AJ, and Isabella;*

*And to the most special person in my life, my wife Patricia, whose love, patience,
encouragement and assistance made this endeavor a reality.*

"The art of medicine is the mastery of chaos"

— R.C. Rollings, Facts and Formulas, Nashville, TE

CONTENTS

FOREWORD

Chronic recurring urticaria (hives) and angioedema (swelling) present difficult challenges for healthcare professionals. Identification of the causes in individual cases is time consuming and difficult, in part because the causes are multiple and extend across almost all medical disciplines. As a result, the simplest approach to treating these conditions may be to accept symptomatic treatment until remission occurs. This approach, although useful in some cases, may result in delay in the identification of serious or non-serious causes that can sometimes be removed or treated without using potentially harmful drugs such as systemic steroids.

There is a lack of useful educational tools to learn about these conditions, both for patients and healthcare professionals. Handouts are notoriously too general and not very helpful for patients. Likewise, healthcare professionals must seek assistance by reading textbook chapters on these conditions, which may not provide practical approaches to everyday problems encountered in clinical practice. Moreover, the recently published practice parameter guidelines for the diagnosis and treatment of urticaria and angioedema may provide useful directions, but are sometimes confusing to healthcare professionals who may not be familiar with the subject.

Dr. Wanderer presents a team approach that defines an active role for the patient in identifying possible causative agents and events. In fact, patients using this approach may be able to identify possible triggers and causes of their symptoms. In addition, there are practical algorithmic guidelines for healthcare professionals, including the differential diagnoses and laboratory tests that may be useful in evaluating patients. This convenient organization is educational for patients and healthcare professionals and should facilitate identification of causes of urticaria and angioedema as well as provide assistance in recommending effective treatments.

This is more than a "how to" book. It is an up-to-date presentation of mechanisms and physiology of urticaria and angioedema and it is arranged in a practical format. Its novelty is that it encourages collaboration between the appropriate people, namely the patient, the healthcare professional and allergy and/or dermatology specialists.

Charles H. Kirkpatrick, M.D.
Professor of Medicine
University of Colorado School of Medicine
Denver, CO

PREFACE:

OBJECTIVES AND HOW TO USE THIS BOOK

EXPLANATION OF TERMINOLOGY

A primary purpose of this book is to improve and standardize the evaluation and treatment of hives and swelling with an approach that encourages collaboration between patients and healthcare professionals. An equally important objective is to empower patients with knowledge and understanding regarding the diagnosis and treatment of these conditions.

In medical literature, **hives** are referred to as **urticaria** and **swelling** as **angioedema**. As you will learn, hives (urticaria) and swelling (angioedema) can be confused with many conditions. When I use the term "hives", I am specifically referring to urticaria as defined by the clinical criteria in chapter 2. Similarly, when I use the term "swelling", I am referring to angioedema, also defined in chapter 2.

Please note that it is possible for hives to occur with or without swelling and for swelling to occur with or without hives. Thus, "hives and/or swellings" are often referred to as "H/S".

The book is divided into three sections, the first providing basic information for patients and healthcare professionals, the second for patients and the last one for healthcare professionals.

Section 1: For patients and optional for healthcare professionals.
- The **Introduction** discusses background information on hives and swelling.
- **Chapter 1** answers common questions regarding hives and swelling.

- **Chapter 2** provides the clinical criteria to establish, with reasonable certainty, if patients are experiencing hives (urticaria) and/or swelling (angioedema).

Section 2: For patients.

- **Chapters 3 and 4** provide workbook exercises for patients.
  - The first exercise is to photograph the hives and/or swelling. This is important because skin symptoms change in appearance and may not be present during scheduled visits with healthcare professionals.
  - The second exercise is to determine whether skin symptoms disappear within a defined time period. Hives (urticaria) characteristically disappear within 24 to 36 hours, and swelling (angioedema) almost always resolves within 72 hours.
  - The third exercise is to complete a detailed history questionnaire that may provide information pertinent to uncovering the cause of the hives and/or swelling.

Section 3: For healthcare professionals.

- **Chapter 5** provides diagnostic recommendations based upon integration of information from the patient's workbook and the physical examination.
- **Chapter 6** discusses treatment strategies for hives and/or swelling.
- **Chapter 7** provides suggestions for evaluation and treatment of hives and/or swelling that are difficult to diagnose and manage.

Some discussions and commentary are repeated in section 3 because different symptoms may be manifestations of the same disease process. For example, puffiness around the eyes, dry skin, and fatigue may all be caused by hypothyroidism secondary to autoimmune thyroiditis. Consequently, discussions and laboratory recommendations are sometimes repeated.

This book is not intended to replace the medical judgment of healthcare professionals and should not be viewed as a medical resource that must be followed in a literal sense in order to arrive at an accurate diagnosis and proper treatment strategy. Rather, it should be considered a means for the exchange of information between patients and healthcare professionals and an information resource that may assist healthcare professionals in the diagnosis and treatment of these conditions. The use of the book should improve diagnostic and treatment success for patients and increase the professional satisfaction of healthcare professionals.

THIS BOOK CAN BE USED BY:

- **Patients** who believe they have hives or swelling. They should complete the workbook and share the information with their healthcare professional.
- **Healthcare professionals** can advise their patients to complete the workbook section and use this material for recommending diagnostic and treatment options.

Both approaches will save time and make for a standardized, efficient and focused interaction between patients and healthcare professionals. Improved collaboration increases the chances of achieving diagnostic and treatment success.

Finally, I would like to emphasize that the evaluation and treatment of chronic hives and swelling requires a "team approach" involving patient, healthcare professional, and specialists (board certified allergists-clinical immunologists, and dermatologists) who can provide added expertise with their academic knowledge, judgment and clinical experience.

SECTION 1:

FOR PATIENTS AND HEALTHCARE PROFESSIONALS

INTRODUCTION

THE MYSTERY AND MISERY OF HIVES

My interest in hives began with a personal experience. I do not have a history of allergies, so I was surprised one morning when I awakened with hives. My first thought, which is typical of hive patients, was that I had developed an allergy to a food or food additive. I treated myself with over-the-counter antihistamines, but the hives persisted and worsened over the next few days. I sought advice from a colleague who was a professor of infectious diseases and mentioned that I had just returned from a vacation in South America. He confirmed the rash was hives and immediately placed me in an isolation ward with the tentative diagnosis of hepatitis, possibly acquired during my South American trip. I was surprised by this possibility, as I was not jaundiced and felt healthy, except for the extremely itchy hives. I entered isolation to protect others from exposure to the disease, in the event his diagnosis was correct. On the seventh day of isolation, the hives disappeared abruptly. The professor, still concerned, requested that I remain in the hospital for a few more days. On the tenth day, I became jaundiced and quite ill with hepatitis, requiring an additional month of hospitalization.

The professor knew something I had not been taught nor experienced, namely that hives are not always a benign or harmless condition, but on occasion, may be a symptom of a more serious, underlying disease. At the time I developed this condition, there was very little information available to explain the association of hives with hepatitis. A decade later, immunology researchers discovered the mechanism that explains how hives can be caused by viral hepatitis. This experience taught me to appreciate the mystery and misery of hives.

Another experience with hives reinforced my decision to choose allergy and immunology as a career specialty. I evaluated a young woman with a history of swelling, hives, and shock, after exposure to cold water. I had never heard of a clinical disorder in which sensitivity to cold temperature caused these symptoms, but her history was very convincing. She had experienced unconsciousness on two occasions while swimming in a lake, and during these episodes, her torso and head became covered with hives. I confirmed that she was sensitive to cold temperature by placing a glass filled with ice cubes on her forearm for about five minutes. After I removed the cold glass, a hive developed that was the size and shape of the bottom of the glass. In addition, placing her hand in a container filled with ice cubes and water caused her entire hand to swell. I focused my research on this problem and discovered that patients with this condition, called acquired cold urticaria, develop abnormal immune responses that cause these symptoms. Once again, I was impressed that hives can be a symptom of a more serious disease.

There are many other examples of hives that are associated with serious disorders. Hives may be the initial manifestation of a systemic reaction (anaphylaxis) to an allergen, such as a bee sting, or from ingesting tree nuts, shellfish and fish. Anaphylactic symptoms may subsequently develop, such as difficulty swallowing, shortness of breath, unconsciousness, shock and possibly death. In this scenario, hives or swelling may precede the onset of a systemic allergic response that requires immediate, life-saving medical attention.

Hives has become a popular term applied to a variety of rashes. It has been confused with eczema, poison ivy, psoriasis, heat rash, insect bites, viral rashes, acne, and even just "itchiness" of the skin. Similarly, other conditions can be confused with swelling (angioedema), such as trauma, fluid overload, blocked veins, obesity, and low thyroid conditions. One of the objectives of this book is to help patients know if they are really experiencing hives (urticaria) or swelling (angioedema).

If you have hives, you are not alone. It is estimated that one out of every five persons in the United States experiences at least one episode of hives in their lifetime.

Think about that number. Approximately sixty million people in the United States, almost twice the population of California, experience hives at least once during their lifetime. Even if the actual number is over-estimated by fifty percent because of inaccurate or mistaken diagnoses, thirty million remains an impressive number. Approximately 5% of these patients may experience symptoms from six weeks up to two years or longer. This suggests that 1.5 million individuals in the United States experience chronic hives.

Self-help health books often refer to hives as just an annoying, itchy problem. These descriptions understate the misery associated with these symptoms. Unless you have experienced hives, it is difficult to appreciate the effect they may have on your life. Wearing ordinary clothing can aggravate symptoms, and patients frequently describe sleeplessness due to constant itching. Middle-of-the-night attempts to control itching by sitting in a bathtub filled with water and oatmeal flakes are representative of the extreme efforts patients make to relieve their symptoms. Some patients describe their disappointment with failures of antihistamine treatments that make them feel tired or behave like "zombies". Sedating antihistamines can also be responsible for accidents and injuries. Patients occasionally describe a sense of isolation and self-consciousness, and wonder if people avoid them because their symptoms appear to be contagious. The economic impacts of chronic hives are not fully appreciated, such as indirect costs associated with reduction of employee efficiency, work absenteeism and the significant costs of medical care and medications.

Patients often feel frightened, neglected, frustrated and sometimes angry, because the underlying causes of their symptoms are infrequently diagnosed. Consequently, they may seek alternative healthcare options, such as herbal treatments, homeopathic therapy, holistic approaches, chiropractic care, megavitamins, animal hormone extracts, anti-yeast regimens, naturopathic food allergy testing, oral drops containing foods or chemicals, and countless other unconventional diagnostic and treatment approaches. There is a passage on hives in a holistic textbook called *The Complete Guide to Natural Healing* that underscores my concerns with alternative approaches. It states "hives are the body's effort to eliminate toxins that have temporarily overloaded the liver and kidneys and thus have shunted to the skin surface in the hope of eliminating such waste products through the skin pores…." "The first thing to do is to take these burdens off the blood cleansing organs and systems and boost the eliminative organs especially the large intestine. If constipated take a laxative and then promote healthy elimination through the bowels." These statements have no scientific foundation, and more importantly, frequent rectal-colonic cleansing using laxatives could result in irregular heart rhythms, seizures, and even shock from electrolyte and fluid imbalance. The use of this approach would be particularly dangerous for hive patients with chronic medical conditions, such as diabetes, cardiac and kidney disease. Alternative therapies and methods are not routinely subjected to scientific scrutiny to prove their effectiveness and safety, and there is no legal requirement to test them in accordance with the Food and Drug Administration (FDA) guidelines. More significantly, exploring alternative care may delay the recognition and treatment of a serious underlying medical condition.

Even though conventional medicine does not understand the cause of hives in most patients, the encouraging news is that major advances in medical science have identified mechanisms that cause some of these conditions. Some hives and swelling are caused by allergic mechanisms of the immune system, while other causes are non-allergic, such as infectious illnesses, cancer, thyroid disorders, immune system abnormalities and genetic or hereditary mechanisms.

My background is founded in evidence-based medicine, which accepts diagnostic approaches and therapies based upon objective, scientific observations, data and statistical confirmation. Most of this text has scientific support. When I introduce personal observations, they are printed in *italic script*.

I decided to write a book on hives to help meet the needs of patients and healthcare professionals. Hopefully, this book will provide patients with knowledge and skills to improve observation of their hives and/or swelling. Their improved observations should assist healthcare professionals consider appropriate diagnostic options, tests, and treatment recommendations.

CHAPTER 1

LEARNING ABOUT HIVES (URTICARIA) AND SWELLING (ANGIOEDEMA)

I recommend reading the questions and answers in sequential order to understand the medical terms as they are introduced and defined.

- What are hives and swelling?
- Why is it difficult to find the cause of hives and/or swelling?
- Is there a common mechanism that causes hives and/or swelling?
- Why do hives and/or swelling remain for a short time in some individuals, while other patients experience symptoms for longer periods, sometimes months or years?
- Can the duration of chronic hives and/or swelling be predicted?
- Why aren't antihistamines completely effective in treating hives and/or swelling?
- How can you determine whether foods, additives, dyes, preservatives, or undetected allergens are causing hives and/or swelling?
- What role do psychological factors play in causing hives and/or swelling?

WHAT ARE HIVES AND SWELLING?

Urticaria is the medical term used to describe itchy, superficial swellings of the skin, otherwise referred to as **hives, wheals** or **welts**. The word is derived from stinging nettle plants belonging to the Urtica genus of plants that can induce hives on direct contact. Urticaria involves superficial swelling of the skin, while **angioedema** refers to swelling inside anatomical compartments located beneath the skin's surface. The word angioedema can be broken into two words of Greek origin, namely, "angos" meaning vessels such as blood vessels, and "oidema" meaning swelling. The involvement of blood vessels in swelling is explained later in this chapter. Angioedema can affect defined anatomical regions, such as lips, fingers, hands, feet, genital organs, and can also involve the mouth, tongue, throat, upper respiratory tract around the trachea (windpipe), and the intestinal tract.

Another rare term used in the medical literature to describe angioedema is angioneurotic edema. The term includes the word "neurotic", suggesting that swelling has a neurological or neurotic cause. This term is rarely used in current medical literature as there are no evidence-based data to support the position that hives and/or swellings are primarily caused by neurological or neurotic mechanisms.

WHY IS IT DIFFICULT TO FIND THE CAUSE OF HIVES AND/OR SWELLING?

Most experts claim they can identify the cause in only one out of every five to ten patients. Despite this discouraging statistic, research discoveries have led to a better understanding of some mechanisms that cause these conditions. Examples of important research discoveries include: (1) the detection and measurement of allergic antibodies (IgE) to foods, animals, etc., that may cause hives and/or swelling; (2) the quantitative measurement of an enzyme (beta tryptase) in the blood, that if elevated, signifies a systemic, allergic reaction is responsible for hives and/or swelling; (3) a recent discovery suggesting there may be an association of thyroid inflammation with these conditions; (4) evidence that viral hepatitis and other viruses sometimes cause hives; and (5) research suggesting inherited traits may be responsible for some hive and/or swelling conditions. Despite these advances, medicine remains limited in the capacity to understand and identify all of the causes of hives and/or swelling.

IS THERE A COMMON MECHANISM THAT CAUSES HIVES AND/OR SWELLING?

Understanding hives and/or swelling requires a discussion of basic biology. **Mast cells** located in the skin and other organ tissues are primarily involved in the development of these symptoms. Other cells and components of the immune system are also involved in causing these conditions. However, for this discussion, I will focus on the most prominent cell type responsible for the development of these symptoms, namely the mast cell. Mast cells contain and manufacture chemicals referred to as **mediators**, such as **histamine, leukotrienes, prostaglandins, and platelet activating factor**. Most hives develop when mediators cause leakage of plasma (water, electrolytes such as sodium and potassium, and protein) through the walls of small blood vessels into the skin. Redness, which occurs when mediators dilate small blood vessels, surrounds the wheal. Swelling occurs when the mediators released from mast cells cause fluid to leak into anatomical compartments located beneath the skin's surface or inside internal organs.

Mediators are released from mast cells for a variety of reasons. Some mechanisms are truly **allergic**, meaning the cause is induced by an allergen, such as food protein or bee venom from a bee sting. A good example of allergic sensitivity is the response to a stinging insect, such as a honey bee. Usually, no clinical symptoms appear the first time a person is stung. The patient's immune system is stimulated to form allergic **antibodies** (proteins formed by the immune system in response to foreign substances) to the bee venom over a period of several months following the initial sting. These allergic antibodies are referred to as IgE antibodies. Following subsequent stings by the same species of insect, or a closely-related species, the venom may access the bloodstream, allowing it to circulate throughout the body and combine to bee venom specific **IgE** antibodies that are attached to mast cells.

Through a series of biochemical events, mast cells release mediators into the skin and the bloodstream, which may cause swelling, hives, and possibly, systemic shock **(anaphylaxis)**.

It is important to mention that not all hives and/or swelling are caused by allergic mechanisms. There are in fact, **non-allergic immune mechanisms** and **non-immune mechanisms** that can induce hives and/or swelling.

Non-allergic immune mechanisms refer to mechanisms involving the immune system that do not cause the production of allergic IgE antibodies. Some non-allergic immune mechanisms may involve classes of antibodies other than IgE. Bacteria, viruses and other infectious organisms can be immobilized by combining with non-allergic antibodies. In turn, these antibodies and infectious organisms combine with a class of proteins in the immune system called **complement**. When this occurs, complement can break down into smaller units called **anaphylatoxins**, which in turn cause the release of chemical mediators from mast cells. The end result is the induction of hives and/or swelling. One clinical example of a non-allergic immune mechanism is an illness called **serum sickness**. This is a serious illness in which patients develop fever, joint pains, hives, and sometimes swelling. Serum sickness may be caused by infections, such as viral hepatitis, and by abnormal immune reactions to antibiotics, such as sulfa and penicillin. In the introduction, I described my own experience with hives which was the result of serum sickness caused by viral hepatitis.

Autoimmunity represents another non-allergic immune mechanism which may cause hives and/or swelling. Autoimmune mechanisms refer to disease states in which individuals develop antibodies to their own cells, tissues and proteins. These antibodies are called **autoantibodies** and belong to classes of antibodies that are different from IgE. Examples of systemic autoimmune diseases that are occasionally associated with hives and/or swelling include rheumatoid arthritis and lupus erythematosus otherwise known as "lupus". There is evidence that some patients with chronic hives exhibit abnormal regulation of an immune pathway, a phenomenon that is also characteristic of systemic autoimmune disorders. This finding supports the theory that chronic hives are occasionally caused by autoimmune mechanisms. In fact, 30% to 40% of patients with chronic hives have autoantibodies to molecules in their blood **(IgE)** and/or to molecules on the surface of mast cells (docking stations for IgE molecules, referred to as **IgE receptors**). It is speculated that autoantibodies, with the help of the complement system, may stimulate the continuous release of mediators from mast cells. The effects of mediators, in turn, cause leakage of plasma and inflammation, which leads to the formation of hives and/or swelling.

Non-immune mechanisms refer to causes of hives and/or swelling that do not involve the immune system. Medications, such as codeine, morphine and some antibiotics, can release mediators by their direct action on mast cells. As a result, symptoms can occur the first time an individual receives these medications. Almost everyone receiving a superficial skin injection of codeine for the first time will develop a localized hive response. This is very different from allergic IgE immune responses, which normally do not cause symptoms following the first exposure to an allergen.

Venoms from snakes, insects, sea urchins and toxins from nettle plants are capable of causing mediator release from mast cells due to the direct action of the venoms/toxins on mast cells. This mechanism explains why localized, and sometimes generalized hives occur the first time someone is bitten by a venomous snake or touches a nettle plant.

Aspirin, ibuprofen, naprosyn and similar medications called **NSAIDS (non steroidal anti-inflammatory drugs)** can induce hives and/or swelling through non-immune mechanisms. These medications can also worsen existing symptoms. Consequently, I advise all patients with hives and/or swelling to avoid NSAIDs. It is not unusual for an individual to take these medications unsuspectingly in over-the-counter medications, such as in Alka-Seltzer® or Empirin®. For this reason patients should recognize aspirin by its chemical name, acetylsalicylic acid. This is another example of why all medications, whether prescription, over-the-counter, herbal, naturopathic etc., need to be included in histories as part of hive and swelling evaluations.

In summary, after reading this information you should have a better appreciation of the many different mechanisms that may induce hives and/or swelling and understand why the causes of these symptoms are elusive and difficult to identify.

WHY DO HIVES AND/OR SWELLING REMAIN FOR A SHORT TIME IN SOME INDIVIDUALS, WHILE OTHERS EXPERIENCE SYMPTOMS FOR LONGER PERIODS, SOMETIMES MONTHS OR YEARS?

Hives and/or swelling are classified into two groups, based on the duration of the symptoms. Hives and/or swelling lasting six weeks or less are called **acute**. If they persist or recur for more than six weeks, they are referred to as **chronic**. Acute hives are commonly caused by allergic sensitivity to an allergen, such as peanuts or from a bee sting. In these examples, acute hives and/or swelling occur when mediators are released from mast cells after the allergen combines with allergic IgE antibodies attached to mast cells. Acute hives and/or swelling usually disappear once the allergen is eliminated from the body.

Medicine now has an improved understanding of *how* hives and/or swelling may become chronic. During the acute stage, mediators such as histamine, are released into the skin or into deep anatomical compartments beneath the skin through allergic and non-allergic immune mechanisms. Certain mediators attract **inflammatory cells (types of white blood cells)** from the bloodstream into the region where the hives and/or swelling are forming. When inflammatory cells arrive, they release new mediators that in turn cause more histamine release from mast cells. Additionally, other kinds of mediators are released into the region. These newly-generated mediators attract more inflammatory cells into the region causing more mediator release, and the process continues to amplify, not unlike an uncontrolled nuclear chain reaction. The end result is hives and/or swelling persist or recur over a protracted period, becoming chronic for months and even years. The process continues until something turns it off internally or anti-inflammatory medications, such as steroids, are introduced to suppress the response.

More recently, research suggests a plausible explanation of *why* chronic hives develop in some patients without an identifiable cause. The research indicates 30% to 40% of patients with chronic hives have antibodies to IgE molecules in their blood and/or to IgE receptors on the surface of mast cells. As mentioned earlier in this chapter, these antibodies are called autoantibodies. It is speculated that autoantibodies, with the help of the complement system, may stimulate the continuous release of mediators from mast cells, which in turn, attract inflammatory cells to the affected region, causing ongoing, chronic hives. There is no known explanation for the appearance of autoantibodies in cases of chronic hives, but this finding provides an explanation of why hives may continue without an identifiable external cause.

CAN THE DURATION OF CHRONIC HIVES AND/OR SWELLING BE PREDICTED?

There is currently no accurate method to predict the duration and outcome of chronic hives and/or swelling. The outcome is best predicted if an underlying disease can be recognized and effectively treated.

Several groups of researchers have done retrospective evaluations of patients with chronic hives and/or swelling of unknown causes. Their findings have been quoted in the allergy and dermatology literature and are the only data available to predict the outcome of these conditions. Based on this data, the following information can be used to predict outcomes:

- 50 % of patients with chronic hives of unknown origin have symptoms for an average duration of 3 to 5 years. Twenty percent (20%) of such patients continue to have symptoms for more than 20 years.
- Patients with more severe hives and/or swelling are less likely to resolve within five years.
- Hive patients with or without swelling seem to have similar outcomes.

Unfortunately these data do not foretell the real story, since many patients with chronic hives and/or swelling have symptoms that persist beyond predicted durations.

WHY AREN'T ANTIHISTAMINES COMPLETELY EFFECTIVE IN TREATING HIVES AND/OR SWELLING?

Antihistamines, as the name suggests, are medications that interfere in the biologic action of histamine, the major mediator released from mast cells. Histamine exerts its biologic effect by binding to docking sites **(histamine receptors)** in the skin. Antihistamines also attach to these receptors, and thus interfere with histamine's ability to exert its physiological effect.

There are basically four reasons why antihistamines do not completely suppress hives and/or swelling.

- First, the efficiency with which antihistamines interfere with the action of histamine depends on their ability to block all the histamine receptors in the skin. This does not usually occur with the recommended doses of prescribed antihistamines. Increasing doses above the recommended range may be associated with side effects. Additionally, the majority of antihistamines can only block one type of histamine receptor, called the H1 receptor. Histamine molecules can also exert their effect through another type of unblocked histamine receptor (the H2 receptor) located in the skin.

- Secondly, antihistamines cannot block the action of other hive-producing mediators, such as leukotrienes, chemokines, kinins, prostaglandins, and platelet activating factor. These mediators appear while an allergic reaction progresses and can prolong the inflammatory process in chronic hives and/or swelling.

- The third reason is antihistamines have minimal or no anti-inflammatory effect. As described previously in this chapter, inflammatory cells migrate into the region of hive and/or swelling formation, releasing mediators which in turn, cause new hives and/or swelling. Antihistamines do not have significant anti-inflammatory benefits and therefore may not prevent recurring symptoms.

- Finally, some antihistamines, such as diphenhydramine (Benadryl®) and hydroxyzine, (Atarax®), may not completely suppress symptoms because patients may not tolerate the recommended doses due to sedative side effects. Reduced intake may lead to skin concentrations of antihistamines that are low, and thus less effective in blocking the action of histamine. Newer second- and third-generation antihistamines, such as Allegra®, Claritin®, Clarinex®, and Zyrtec®, are tolerated more easily because they generally do not cause significant sedation. Consequently, the reduction in sedative effects with second and third generation antihistamines is associated with better compliance which may be partially responsible for their effectiveness in suppressing hives and/or swelling.

In summary, antihistamines do not completely suppress hives and/or swelling. Knowing that antihistamines have limitations may help patients understand and accept why their symptoms "break through" while they are taking these medications. This is one of the reasons why healthcare professionals continue to experiment with combinations of antihistamines and other medications to achieve suppression of symptoms.

HOW CAN YOU DETERMINE WHETHER FOODS, FOOD ADDITIVES, DYES, PRESERVATIVES, OR UNDETECTED ALLERGENS IN FOOD ARE CAUSING HIVES AND/OR SWELLING?

Some medical literature supports the notion that acute hives and/or swelling can be caused by sensitivity to foods, food additives, or undetected allergens. In general, an acute episode of hives and/or swelling that occurs after the ingestion of a suspect food, such as peanuts or shellfish, can be diagnosed using conventional skin tests or with blood tests, called IgE allergen-specific RAST tests. Unfortunately, this is not the case with chronic hives and/or swelling, as it is extremely difficult to detect a food or food additive that is causing chronic symptoms.

Part of the difficulty with isolating a food as the cause of chronic hives and/or swelling is determining whether testing should be done with a fresh food, a cooked food or a food metabolite. Cooking usually destroys protein and complex carbohydrate allergens in foods, although allergens in certain foods, such as in almonds, can remain stable after cooking. In other circumstances, cooking may actually enhance the allergic potential of a food, such as roasting peanuts. Consequently, even if a food induces hives and/or swelling according to the patient's history, healthcare professionals may not know how the food material should be prepared for testing.

Food allergy skin tests can produce false negative results if the test material does not include the allergen to which the patient may be allergic. Conversely, food skin tests may produce false positive results that inaccurately predict the existence of an allergy. The IgE RAST test is a legitimate blood test that detects IgE antibodies to a food. However, it too has limitations because it can give false negative results due to its inherent lower sensitivity. The best test to detect a relationship between the ingestion of a food and the induction of hives and/or swelling is to perform carefully controlled, oral challenges under medical supervision. Ideally, the healthcare professional performs blind, oral challenges in graduated doses; "blind" meaning the flavor of the food is masked so the patient is unaware of the kind of food being ingested. Amounts of food are increased gradually to prevent a serious allergic reaction.

Further complicating matters is the possibility that foods may occasionally induce hives and/or swelling by alternative immune mechanisms that do not involve the production of allergic IgE antibodies. Unfortunately, these alternative immune responses cannot be detected by conventional food skin tests or by IgE RAST tests.

Identifying the food that induces hives and/or swelling is made difficult by the fact that foods contain additives, preservatives, dyes, other chemicals and undeclared food allergens. Detecting allergic sensitivity to dyes is difficult, although a recent study suggests skin testing may occasionally identify dye sensitivity. An allergy to undeclared food is also difficult to uncover. In some cases, individuals with peanut allergy have experienced severe allergic reactions after eating foods containing undeclared peanut. Another example of an undeclared food is fish albumin, which is used in processing French wines. Additionally, farmers and ranchers add antibiotics, such as tetracycline, penicillin and quinolones to animal feed to reduce infections and enhance growth in livestock. The presence of trace amounts of penicillin is of particular concern because it is a heat-stable molecule that remains unchanged by sterilization of milk products or cooking of meat. It is speculated small amounts of penicillin present in foods could explain the recurrence of hives and/or swelling in persons sensitive to this antibiotic. Similarly, many antibiotics and unknown chemical additives in food products probably play a role in the induction of these symptoms.

Attempts to determine whether food additives and preservatives are causing these conditions can be frustrating. There are numerous chemicals that are added to foods, such as taste enhancers, preservatives, hormones, and antibiotics. Food manufacturers often decline to provide information about additives on the grounds they are trade secrets. Most of these additives are not available to the medical profession for testing, and even if they were, it is difficult to foretell whether testing with these chemicals would provide accurate and predictive information. A new National Organic Rule of the United States Department of Agriculture (USDA) may be helpful in identifying foods that are produced with additives. The labeling of a food must include its classification in one of four categories: 100% ORGANIC designates completely organic food that does not contain non-organic ingredients; "ORGANIC" means at least 95% of the product's ingredients are organic; "MADE WITH ORGANIC INGREDIENTS" signifies at least 70% of the ingredients are organic and that the product contains no sulfites, chemicals that can cause asthma; and "SOME ORGANIC INGREDIENTS" identifies products with less than 70% organic ingredients. This labeling system should be very helpful to individuals who may have hives and/or swelling due to food additives.

Additionally, food biochemists have modified some plants genetically to enhance growth, resist insects and pests, and prevent adverse reactions to weed killers. Advantageous genes from one plant species are transplanted to another species, a process that has been accomplished with commercially available corn, soybeans and tomatoes. Genetically modified plants may cause hives and/or swelling in individuals sensitive to proteins produced by transplanted genes derived from a different plant or animal species. Unfortunately, the FDA does not require labeling food products that are derived from genetically modified plants.

Some healthcare professionals subject their patients to food elimination diets and then add a single fresh food in an attempt to identify foods or food additives that may be the cause of hives and/or swelling. This method has more merit than attempts to identify a food by using expensive, unreliable blood tests. The patient is placed on a diet consisting only of a food supplement that contains completely metabolized (elemental) foods, such as Progestimil®, Tolerex®) and E028Extra (SHS International). After one or two weeks, a single, freshly-made food is added for three to four days, during which the patient monitors the severity of the symptoms for a flare-up. This process is continued until most major foods are added into the diet.

The important point of this discussion is that isolating a food that is causing hives and/or swelling can be extremely difficult. Consequently, patients who believe foods are the cause of their symptoms need to be careful when considering expensive, unreliable tests and treatments that are scientifically unproven. I recommend visiting the Food Allergy and Anaphylaxis Network (www.foodallergy.org) to learn more about the role of food allergy as a cause of hives and/or swelling. This site provides new approaches and research information on this subject.

There are some cautions that need to be emphasized regarding commercially available food tests that claim to accurately detect food allergy. The American Academy of Allergy, Asthma, and Immunology has developed position papers on all but kinesiology testing and declared them to be **invalid** predictors of food allergy:

- **Cytotoxic blood test**: This test is performed by adding a food allergen to a blood specimen and inspecting for white blood cell alteration, which is claimed to be indicative of food allergy.

- **Provocative and neutralization testing by oral administration and injection techniques**: These methods involve the injection of a food allergen subcutaneously (into the skin), or the application of food drops under the tongue, to elicit symptoms corresponding to the patients' complaints. This is followed by the injection or oral drop administration of the same allergen at a weaker strength, presumably to relieve symptoms.

- **Pulse tests**: These tests are based on the unfounded claim that food allergy can be detected by monitoring increases in the pulse rate after the ingestion of a food.

- **Kinesiology testing**: This test is based on the unfounded claim that an allergic reaction to a food can be detected by monitoring changes in muscle strength. The NAET method involves placing a food in the patient's hand and then pushing down on the patient's flexed arm to test for muscle weakness. The patient is claimed to be allergic to the food if arm weakness is detected. There is no position paper on this technique. One can read critically about this unscientific technique by accessing the following site: http://www. chirobase.org/06DD/naet.html.

- **RAST IgG antibodies:** This test is based on the unfounded claim that elevated IgG antibodies to specific foods are indicative of food allergy. In fact, most individuals exhibit positive food IgG RAST tests, and the results do not correlate with clinical evidence of food allergy or other disease states. These tests should not be confused with RAST tests that detect IgE allergic antibodies to foods.

WHAT ROLE DO PSYCHOLOGICAL FACTORS PLAY IN CAUSING HIVES AND/OR SWELLING?

Older medical literature describes angioedema as angioneurotic edema. The term includes the word "neurotic", suggesting that swelling has a neurotic cause. I have spoken to psychiatrists and psychologists about this issue and their position is generally favorable to the hypothesis that psychological factors, such as anxiety, panic reactions, and depression can cause or exacerbate these conditions. Studies measuring anxiety and depression indicate that patients with chronic hives have higher scores for both of these psychological responses, compared to control patients with other skin conditions. Unfortunately, these studies have not answered the key question, namely, whether these psychological responses are the cause or effect of chronic hives and/or swelling.

A few types of hive disorders occur due to abnormal physiologic responses to stress. In one condition, called **adrenergic urticaria**, the redness that typically surrounds commonplace hives is replaced by blanched, white halos. Some researchers believe this condition is caused by the excessive production of adrenalin-like chemicals during stress. Another type of hives associated with stress and increased body heat production is **cholinergic urticaria**. Patients typically develop pinpoint, itchy hives when undergoing stress or when they become overheated during exercise. This condition may reflect an increased sensitivity to chemicals released by the nervous system.

There are also proponents for the negative position on this controversy. *In my informal survey of allergists and other healthcare professionals, many expressed the opinion that psychological factors are not primary causes of chronic hives and/or swelling. More likely, these* symptoms may cause psychological stress in otherwise healthy individuals. Mood changes, panic reactions, depression, and anxiety may occur in individuals with healthy psyches as a consequence of not knowing what is causing their hives and/or swelling, concerns about the possible presence of serious underlying disease, and functional impairment in their daily activities.

In conclusion, there are no evidence-based data to support the suggestion that these conditions have a "neurotic" causation. I recommend treatment of abnormal psychological reactions if it is determined they are responses to hives and/or swelling. This may include the addition of medications to the treatment regime, such as anti-anxiety or anti-depression drugs, and/or the need for psychological counseling.

CHAPTER 2

HOW TO BE SURE PATIENTS ARE EXPERIENCING HIVES (URTICARIA) AND/OR SWELLING (ANGIOEDEMA)

This chapter describes the appearance of hives and swelling and the clinical criteria required for their diagnosis. "Hives" has become a vernacular term for almost all rashes. Consequently, patients often seek an evaluation thinking they are experiencing hives, when in fact, their rash represents an entirely different medical condition. There are also conditions that are confused with swelling. Unfortunately, no tests exist to definitively confirm a diagnosis of hives and/or swelling. The answers to the following questions may assist in the diagnosis of hives and/or swelling:

• What is the appearance of hives (urticaria)?
• What are the clinical criteria to confirm a diagnosis of hives (urticaria)?
• What is the appearance of swelling (angioedema)?
• What are the clinical criteria to confirm a diagnosis of swelling (angioedema)?

Other medical conditions that can be confused with hives and/or swelling are described in Appendix I.

WHAT IS THE APPEARANCE OF HIVES (URTICARIA)?

An example of classic hives, on a small scale, is the swelling and redness resulting from a mosquito bite or bee sting. Insect stings can produce small, itchy, swollen areas that are pale and white or pink. The swelling is commonly referred to as a **wheal** or **welt.** Typically, redness surrounds the outer edges of the welt. Hives can be as small as the diameter of a pencil point or as large as a platter, sometimes joining together to form large areas referred to as "giant urticaria". See figures 1 and 2 in **the color section of the book** to help recognize this condition.

WHAT ARE THE CLINICAL CRITERIA TO CONFIRM A DIAGNOSIS OF HIVES (URTICARIA)?

- In general, hives are very itchy and soft to the touch.
- Hives have a swollen, raised, central area that is pale white or pale pink. This swelling is commonly referred to as a wheal or welt. Sometimes the welt may not be obvious because the affected person's skin is dark. The welt can be made more obvious by spreading the skin in opposite directions outside the margins of the welt.
- A red area surrounds the pale white or pale pink central area.
- The borders of the welt are irregular and jagged shaped.
- Hives characteristically fade within 24 to 36 hours at one location and may reappear at other locations. This is a very important diagnostic feature of hives.

Other medical conditions, such as erythema multiforme, which may be confused with hives (urticaria) are described in Appendix 1.

WHAT IS THE APPEARANCE OF SWELLING (ANGIOEDEMA)?

The appearance of swelling (angioedema) is similar to the traumatic swelling of a boxer's face after a match. Both "trauma-induced swelling" and swelling (angioedema) involve deep anatomical compartments that become filled with fluid. These compartments prevent any type of swelling from extending beyond distinct anatomical boundaries, which is an important defense against infections which could otherwise spread throughout the body. There is a major difference between the fluids that cause swelling in each condition. "Trauma-induced swelling" is caused by the accumulation of blood that results when blood vessels are ruptured. Subsequent black and blue discoloration occurs as blood is broken down and re-absorbed. In contrast, swelling associated with angioedema involves the accumulation of plasma fluid (composed of water, electrolytes, and protein) that has leaked through the walls of small intact blood vessels into deep anatomically defined compartments. A variety of mechanisms that cause swelling (angioedema) are described in **chapter 1**. See figures 3 and 4 in **the color section in this book** to help recognize this condition.

WHAT ARE THE CLINICAL CRITERIA TO CONFIRM
A DIAGNOSIS OF SWELLING (ANGIOEDEMA)?

- Swelling occurs below the skin surface and is confined to defined anatomical compartments, such as an eyelid, lip, ear, hand, finger, foot, toe, tongue and scrotum. It may also involve internal organs, such as the intestinal tract, bladder, reproductive organs, and also the upper respiratory region around the trachea (windpipe).
- Swelling around the tongue and inside the mouth can interfere with swallowing and breathing and is considered a serious medical emergency.
- Swelling may be associated with tenderness and pain. This occurs because swelling is restricted to defined anatomical compartments which do not stretch easily. For this reason, the involvement of a hand, foot or finger can be very painful.

- Swelling may cause abdominal pain and cramps when it involves the intestinal tract.
- Swelling is not associated with itching.
- Swelling typically disappears within 24 to 72 hours, depending on the severity.
- Pushing on a swollen area with a fingertip may leave an indentation for a few seconds.
- Swelling is characteristically asymmetrical. For example, swelling of one hand is not typically associated with a mirror image swelling of the other hand.

Other medical conditions that may be confused with swelling (angioedema), such as lymphedema, are described in Appendix 1.

Please note it is possible for hives to occur with or without swelling and for swelling to occur with or without hives. If your symptoms match the criteria for hives and/or swelling described here, proceed to chapters 3 and 4 and complete the workbook exercises which may help uncover the cause of your symptoms.

SECTION 2:

WORKBOOK FOR

PATIENTS

CHAPTER 3

EXERCISES TO HELP CONFIRM THE PRESENCE OF HIVES (URTICARIA) AND/OR SWELLING (ANGIOEDEMA)

- Take photographs when symptoms are at their peak.
- Take photographs when the symptoms first appear, and then observe whether hives and/or swelling disappear within a period of time consistent with their diagnostic criteria.

EXERCISE #1: TAKE PHOTOGRAPHS AT THE PEAK OF SYMPTOMS.

Purpose:

To capture the appearance of skin symptoms at their peak and to confirm they are actually hives and/or swelling.

Explanation:

More frequently than I would predict, patients arrive for an appointment and no hives and/or swelling are present despite a history of daily symptoms. Ironically, symptoms may reoccur within days after the appointment. I can't explain this phenomenon other than to suspect that anticipation of the visit causes some patients to produce extra stress hormones, such as adrenalin and cortisone, which could temporarily suppress their symptoms.

I recommend obtaining good quality **close up** and **full view** photographs, if possible when the symptoms are at their peak. These photographs will help make a more accurate diagnosis. Photographs will also provide the healthcare professional with a better appreciation of the severity of the symptoms. Antihistamines and steroid medications will alter and suppress the appearance of hives and/or swelling, so it is advisable the photographs be taken when these medications have been discontinued. **These medications should be discontinued *only* on the advice of a healthcare professional**.

ATTACH THE PHOTOGRAPHS OF YOUR
SKIN SYMPTOMS TAKEN AT THEIR PEAK APPEARANCE.

FULL VIEWS (DATE AND TIME)_____

CLOSE UP VIEWS (DATE AND TIME)_____

EXERCISE #2:
2A—OBSERVE WHETHER HIVES (URTICARIA) DISAPPEAR
WITHIN 24 to 36 HOURS
2B—OBSERVE WHETHER SWELLING (ANGIOEDEMA)
DISAPPEARS WITHIN 72 HOURS

Purpose:

To determine whether hives disappear within 24 to 36 hours and whether swelling disappears within 72 hours.

Explanation:

Usually hives disappear at a specific location after 24 to 36 hours and then reappear at a different location. If they remain unchanged at a specific location for more than 24 to 36 hours, there is a distinct possibility the symptoms may not be hives. Swelling should also disappear within 24 to 36 hours, although it may take up to 72 hours to completely resolve. Swelling lasting more than 72 hours is generally not characteristic of angioedema.

Procedure:

This is an important exercise to complete accurately. Photographs should be taken when the hives and/or swelling **first appear**, and then, **24 to 36 hours later**, for hives, and **72 hours later**, for swelling. Circle one to three different hives (**Exercise 2A**), and if present, one area of swelling (**Exercise 2B**) and number each area with an indelible marker. Note the time of day, record the size of the hives and/or swelling and attach the photographs of each skin location in this workbook. Record the same information for hives 24 to 36 hours after they appeared, and attach the photographs in the spaces provided. Similarly, if you are experiencing swelling, record the same information 72 hours after the swelling appears, and attach the photograph in the space provided.

Antihistamines and steroid medications will alter and suppress the appearance of hives and/or swelling, so ideally, the photographs should be obtained when these medications have been discontinued. **These medications should be discontinued** *only* **on the advice of a healthcare professional.**

BASELINE OBSERVATIONS

EXERCISE 2A—HIVES:
TAKE PHOTOGRAPHS WHEN THE SYMPTOMS FIRST APPEAR,
AND THEN 24 TO 36 HOURS LATER, AND ATTACH IN THE
SPACES PROVIDED BELOW, WITH THE INFORMATION REQUESTED.

Hive location #1:
- Date and time of day: _____
- Location: _____
- Measure vertical and horizontal diameters (also record the unit of measurement, i.e. mm; ⅛ inch):
  — Vertical (Height) diameter: _____
  — Horizontal (Width) diameter: _____
- Photograph a **close view** of hive location #1.

Attach photograph of hive location #1 here.

Hive location #2:

- Date and time of day: _____
- Location: _____
- Measure vertical and horizontal diameters (also record the unit of measurement, i.e. mm; ⅛ inch):
  — Vertical (Height) diameter: _____
  — Horizontal (Width) diameter: _____
- Photograph a **close view** of hive location #2.

Attach photograph of hive location #2 here.

Hive location #3:

- Date and time of day: _____
- Location: _____
- Measure vertical and horizontal diameters (also record the unit of measurement, i.e. mm; ⅛ inch):
  — Vertical (Height) diameter: _____
  — Horizontal (Width) diameter: _____
- Photograph a **close view** of hive location #3.

Attach photograph of hive location #3 here.

CONTINUATION OF EXERCISE 2A:
OBSERVE THE SAME HIVES AND RECORD 24 TO 36 HOURS LATER

Hive #1 (24 to 36 hours later):

- Date and time of day: _____
- Location: _____
- Measure vertical and horizontal diameters (also record the unit of measurement, i.e. mm; ⅛ inch):
  — Vertical (Height diameter: _____
  — Horizontal (Width) diameter:_____
- Photograph a **close view** of hive location #1.

Attach photograph of hive #1 (24 to 36 hours later).

Hive #2 (24 to 36 hours later):

- Date and time of day: _____
- Location: _____
- Measure vertical and horizontal diameters (also record the unit of measurement, i.e. mm; ⅛ inch):
  — Vertical (Height) diameter: _____
  — Horizontal (Width) diameter: _____
- Photograph a **close view** of hive location #2.

Attach photograph of hive #2 (24 to 36 hours later).

Hive #3 (24 to 36 hours later):

- Date and time of day: _____
- Location: _____
- Measure vertical and horizontal diameters (also record the unit of measurement, i.e. mm; ⅛ inch):
  — Vertical (Height diameter: _____
  — Horizontal (Width) diameter: _____
- Photograph a **close view** of hive location #3.

Attach photograph of hive #3 (24 to 36 hours later).

EXERCISE 2B. SWELLING:
TAKE PHOTOGRAPHS OF THE SWELLING WHEN IT FIRST APPEARS,
AND WHEN IT DISAPPEARS WITHIN 72 HOURS.
ATTACH THE PHOTOGRAPHS IN THE SPACES PROVIDED BELOW,
WITH THE INFORMATION REQUESTED.

Swelling:
- Date and time of day: _____
- Location: _____
- Measure vertical and horizontal diameters (also record the unit of measurement, i.e. mm; ⅛ inch):
  — Vertical (Height diameter: _____
  — Horizontal (Width) diameter: _____
- Photograph a **close view** of swelling.

Attach photograph of swelling here.

CONTINUATION OF EXERCISE 2B:
OBSERVE THE SAME SWELLING AND RECORD
THE TIME IT DISAPPEARS:

Swelling (up to 72 hours later):

- Date and time of day: _____
- Location: _____
- Measure vertical and horizontal diameters (also record the unit of measurement, i.e. mm; ⅛ inch):
  — Vertical (Height diameter: _____
  — Horizontal (Width) diameter diameter: _____
- Photograph a **close view** of swelling.

Attach photograph of swelling (72 hours later).

The next exercise requires completion of the history questionnaire in chapter 4 which may provide important clues to understanding the cause of hives and/or swelling. Please proceed to chapter 4.

CHAPTER 4

HISTORY QUESTIONNAIRE

Despite all of the technological advances in medicine, the ability to identify the underlying causes of hives and/or swelling relies primarily on information derived from a history. The usefulness of a history depends on two factors; first, the accuracy of observations provided by the patient and secondly, whether the appropriate questions are asked by healthcare professionals. The purpose of this chapter is to utilize an improved, standardized patient history questionnaire that will provide healthcare professionals with the information they need to help recognize causes of hives and/or swelling.

The history questionnaire deals with general symptoms that may appear to be unrelated to hives and/or swelling, such as fatigue, weight gain/loss, and fever. Although these symptoms are non-specific, they may provide direction to unsuspected medical conditions. In addition, detailed questions about most organ systems have been included, since hives and/or swelling can be manifestations of generalized, systemic disorders.

PLEASE CIRCLE THE DESCRIPTIONS THAT APPLY TO YOU AND FILL IN THE ANSWERS TO THE QUESTIONS RELATED TO YOUR SYMPTOMS. HIVES (URTICARIA) AND/OR SWELLINGS (ANGIOEDEMA) ARE USUALLY ABBREVIATED AS H/S IN THE QUESTIONNAIRE.

The numbers in bold face following the questions are for the healthcare professional to consider possible diagnosis and treatment suggestions in Section 3.

A. General questions

■ Do you think you are experiencing? **(#1)**
  - Hives
  - Swelling
  - Both hives and swelling

■ How long have you had the symptoms? **(#2)**
  - Less than 6 weeks
  - 6 weeks to 1 yr
  - More than 1 yr (duration _____)
    ○ Date you first experienced H/S _____
    ○ Date you last experienced H/S _____

■ What time of day do the symptoms occur? **(#3)**
  - Daytime
  - Nighttime
  - Both daytime and nighttime

■ How often do the symptoms occur? **(#4)**
  - A daily occurrence
  - Intermittent
    ○ # of times per week ____)
    ○ # times monthly _____)
    ○ Less than monthly (# times __ every __ months)

- Which part of your body was first affected with H/S? **(#5)** _____

- Does H/S occur more frequently during a particular season of the year? **(#6)**

  Winter   Spring   Summer   Fall

- In your opinion, have your symptoms changed since they started? **(#7)**

  Worsened   Unchanged   Improved

B. Are you experiencing any of the following symptoms with H/S? Please circle any of the following symptoms you experience and answer the related questions.

- General:
  - Fatigue **(#8)**
  - Fever **(#9)**
  - Unexplained weight gain
    Amount gained _____, over how long? _____ **(#10)**
  - Unexplained weight loss
    Amount of weight loss _____, over how long?_____ **(#11)**
  - Emotional symptoms (anxiety, mood swings, panic reactions, depression) **(#12)**
    ○ Do stressful situations cause you to develop hives?

      Yes   No

- Skin
  - Dry skin **(#13)**
  - Bruising easily **(#14)**
  - Unusual amount of hair loss **(#15)**

- Face
  - Tenderness over face **(#16)**
  - Discolored nasal discharge **(#17)**

- Eyes
  - Puffiness around eyes   **(#18)**

- Throat
  - Sore throat, difficulty swallowing, hoarseness **(#19)**
  - Cold sores   **(#20)**
  - Painful teeth, gum disease **(#21)**

- Bones and Joints
  - Joint pain   **(#22)**
  - Joint swelling **(#23)**
  - Bone pain **(#23A)**
  - Frequent bone fractures: How many _____   **(#24)**

- Respiratory Symptoms **(#25)**
  - Chronic cough
  - Shortness of breath
  - Wheezing

- Gastrointestinal Symptoms **(#26); (#26A to #26F)**
  - Abdominal pain   Duration _____, and location _____
  - Nausea
  - Vomiting
  - Diarrhea
  - Blood in stools

- Symptoms involving the Urinary and Reproductive Systems **(#27); (#27A to #27H)**
  - History of H/S coinciding with menstrual cycle
  - Burning sensation with urination
  - Sharp, low back pains
  - Increased frequency of urination
  - Decreased frequency of urination
  - History of blood in urine

- History of sexually transmitted disease. Specify_____
- History of AIDS or risk factors for AIDS (sexual activities outside of mono-gamous relationship, use of illegal intravenous drugs, blood transfusions) Specify _____

  _____

■ Muscle and Nerve Symptoms **(#28);(#28A to #28E)**
  - Muscle weakness, if so, where? _____
  - Muscle pains, if so, where? _____
  - Decreased or abnormal skin sensation. Explain: _____

  _____

C. Circle the situations that trigger or worsen your H/S symptoms, and answer the related questions.

■ Rubbing or scratching your skin **(#29)**
  - Are there other members of your family who have H/S after rubbing or scratching **(#36A)**?

    Yes   No

■ Painful swelling from sustained pressure, such as **(#30)**:
  - Tight clothing (belt, bra, or stockings) causes painful swelling under these garments.
  - Painful swelling of hand(s) after using tools.
  - Standing for long periods, excessive walking or running causes painful swelling of feet.
  - Carrying heavy objects causes painful swelling of shoulders, arms, or hands.
  - Prolonged sitting causes painful swelling of buttocks.
  - List any other activities that cause painful swelling:

  _____

  _____

■ Exposure to sunlight **(#31)**

- Exposure to cold temperatures, swimming or other water sports **(#32)**

- Exercise **(#33)**
  - Are there other members of your family who have H/S after exercise? **(36B)**

    Yes   No

- Bathing or showering in warm or hot water **(#34)**

- Contact with water involving all ranges of water temperature **(#35)**
  - Are there other members of your family who experience H/S following contact with water, regardless of temperature? **(#38A)**

    Yes   No

D. Family history of H/S.

- Are there other members of your family with H/S?

    Yes   No

- If the answer to the last question is yes, list all affected family members who are genetically related to you (blood relatives).

  _____

  _____

- If there are other members of your family with H/S, circle any of the following triggers or conditions associated with their H/S:
  - Vibration **(#36)**
  - Cold Exposure **(#37, #38)**
  - Swelling in mouth following dental procedures, unusual swelling from mild injury to a body part or swelling for unknown reasons **(#39)**
  - Affected family members with H/S in combination with deafness and/or kidney disease (nephrosis) **(#40)**
  - Swelling occurs only in females taking estrogens, birth control pills or during pregnancy **(#41)**

- Exercise **(#36B)**
- Contact with water involving all ranges of temperature **(#38A)**
- Scratching or rubbing skin **(#36A)**

E. If H/S increases at work, at home or during recreational activities, answer the following questions:

■ State your occupation and the tasks you perform in this occupation:

_____

■ List occupational exposures you suspect may be associated with or may cause H/S: _____

■ **(#42)** Do you work in the healthcare profession?

Yes   No

■ **(#43)** Are you exposed to latex at work?

Yes   No

■ **(#44)** Are you exposed to animals at work, such as in veterinarian clinics, farming or other situations?

Yes   No

■ If H/S occurs at home, list details, such as time of day, where you were in the house, and what you were doing.

Specify: _____

_____

- **(#45)** Does H/S occur during exposure to animals?

Yes   No

- **(#46)** Does H/S occur while working with arts and crafts?

Yes   No

■ If H/S occurs during or after recreational activities, please specify:

_____

• **(#47)** Does H/S occur during or after water sports?

Yes   No

• **(#48)** Does H/S occur during or after exercise, jogging or other sports activities? If yes, please specify: _____

• **(#49)** Does H/S occur with weight-lifting?

• Other recreational activities associated with H/S:

_____

F. **Medication history (#50):**

In the space below, list all the medications: (1) you are taking since the onset of H/S; (2) you were taking during the month prior to onset of H/S; and (3) you discontinued after the onset of H/S. The lists should include prescription medications, all over-the-counter medications including herbs, vitamins, and health supplements. Include medications delivered by all modes of administration, including oral medications; medications received by injection including vaccinations and antibiotics; rectally or vaginally, such as suppositories or douches; medications applied topically to the skin such as patches, ointments, creams, gels; nasal sprays or drops; oral sprays; drops and/or ointments applied to the eyes or ears. **Make copies of the labels with the contents of each product you were, or are using and, if possible, take all your medications, supplements, etc., to your healthcare professional.**

_____

_____

_____

_____

_____

_____

_____

_____

- List the names of all cosmetics, shampoos, hair conditioners, soaps, detergents, spot removers, fabric softeners, dryer sheets (static-reducing laundry products), etc., you are using. **Make copies of the labels with the contents of each product and if possible, bring them with you to your healthcare professional's office.**

_____

_____

_____

_____

G. **History of insect stings. Circle or fill in answers. (#51)**. Please include stings by bees, fire ants, ticks, deer flies and other insects.

- History of present and past insect sting: specify the date of sting(s), the location of sting(s), and the type of insect, if known:

_____

_____

_____

_____

- Have you experienced H/S from insect sting(s)? If yes, specify the date of sting, the type of insect, and the location of sting(s):

_____

H. **Food history. (#52)**:

- Do you suspect food(s) cause or trigger your H/S?:

Yes   No

If yes, please specify:

_____

_____

■ Does H/S occur immediately (within 20 to 30 minutes) after ingestion or contact with a suspect food?

Yes   No

If yes, list the suspect foods:

_____

■ Are symptoms of H/S delayed after ingestion of a suspect food (occurs more than 60 minutes after ingestion of the food)?

Yes   No

If yes, list amount of time that H/S occur after the ingestion of suspect food(s) along with the name of the suspect food(s):

_____

■ Does H/S disappear after elimination of the suspect food from your diet?

Yes   No

■ Does H/S reoccur after re-ingesting the same suspect food?

Yes   No

■ Does H/S occur after you ingest **fresh** preparations of the suspect food(s)?

Yes   No

• Fresh means the food is prepared from the original produce and is not a canned, frozen, or boxed product.

I. **Travel history. (#53)**:

■ Have you traveled to a foreign country within two years prior to the onset of H/S?

Yes   No

If yes, please specify countries and date(s):

_____

■ Have you experienced diarrhea and/or vomiting since foreign travel?

Yes   No

■ Have you ingested water from a well, river, pond, lake or other unpurified water source within one year prior to the onset H/S?

Yes   No

■ Have you received injections or transfusions in a foreign country?

Yes   No

J. Hormone history. Circle situations that may apply to you and answer the related questions. (#54 through #57):

■ Do you notice any of the following symptoms?
  • Enlargement or lumps in front of neck? **(#54, #55, #56)**. Specify details:

  _____

  _____

  • Unexplained weight gain **(#54)**
  • Unexplained weight loss **(#55)**
  • Unusual hair loss **(#54)**
  • Irregular menstrual cycle **(#54)**
  • Dry skin **(#54)**
  • Prominence of eyes **(#55)**
  • Tremors **(# 55)**
  • History of kidney stones **(# 56)**
  • History of frequent bone fractures **(# 56)**
    Specify number of fractures: _____ and bones fractured:

  _____

■ History of thyroid disease
  • High thyroid condition **(#55)**
  • Low thyroid condition **(#54)**

- History of thyroiditis (inflammation of the thyroid sometimes called Hashimoto's thyroiditis) **(#54, #55)**

■ For women: Does H/S correlate with menstrual cycle? **(#57, #57A)**

Yes   No

■ For women: Does **swelling without hives** occur in an inherited pattern that affects only women in your family who are taking estrogens, birth control pills or during pregnancy? **(#57B)**

Yes   No

■ For women: Do H/S occur only during pregnancies? **(#57B, #57C)**

Yes   No

K. History of infections. Circle the situations that may apply to you and answer the questions related to your history of infections occurring with H/S, or symptoms of infections in the past; (#58)

■ History of fever at the time of onset of H/S **(#58,#58A)**. Date when fever started:_____

■ In order to assess your immune system, please list the major infections (pneumonia, sinusitis, ear infections, skin infections such as abscesses, meningitis), treated or not treated, that you have experienced: **(#58, #58B)**

_____

_____

_____

■ History of hepatitis **(#58, #59)**. Date of onset:_____

■ History of jaundice. **(#58, #59)**. Date of onset: _____

■ History of sore throat at the time of onset of H/S. **(#58, #60)**. Date of onset:

_____

- History of "strep" throat documented by throat culture or fast streptococcal test **(#58, #60)** at the time of onset of H/S. Date of onset:_____

- History of infectious mononucleosis. **(#58, #61)**. Date of onset: _____

- History of cold sores.**(#58, #62)**. Date of onset: _____

- History of a chronic wound with or without drainage. **(#58, #63)**. Date of onset: _____

- History of discolored drainage from nose at the time of onset of H/S. **(#58, #64)**. Date of onset:_____

- History of sinus infections.**(#58, #64)**. Date of onset:_____

- History of gum infection, dental abscess. **(#58, #65)**. Date of onset: _____

- History of stomach ulcer **(#58, #66)**. Date of onset: _____

- History of gallstones or gallbladder attacks **(#58, #67)**. Date of onset: _____

- History of fungal infection, such as athlete's foot **(#58,#68)**. Date of onset: _____

- History of skin infection, skin abscess **(#58,#69)**. Date of onset: _____

- History of yeast infection **(#58, #70)**. Date of onset: _____
  Location: _____

- History of bronchitis or pneumonia. **(#58, #71)**. Date of onset: _____

- History of urinary infection **(#58, #72)**. Date of onset:_____

- History of sexual transmitted infection, HIV (AIDS), syphilis, gonorrhea, or other **(#58, #73)**. Date of onset:_____

- History of transfusion **(#58, #74)**. Specify situation and date:

  _____

- Histories of needle stick(s) **(#58, #75).** Specify situation and date:

  _____

L. History of tumors, cancers. Circle the situations that apply to you and answer the related questions. (#76)

- History of recent mass, lump on skin or beneath skin?
  Specify location: _____ Duration:_____

- History of recent lymph node swelling. Specify location(s): _____
  Duration:_____

- History of previously diagnosed cancer.
  Specify: _____

- Recent history of any of the following symptoms:
  - Cough. If yes, give the date of last chest-X-ray:_____
  - Unexplained weight loss
  - Unexplained bleeding at any location. Specify location: _____
  - Unexplained pain or tenderness at any location.
    Specify location: _____ Duration:_____

M. History of direct skin contact with environmental substances that may be associated with H/S. (#77 through #83).

- Does H/S occur during or after skin contact with plants? **(#77)** Specify type of plant: _____

- Does H/S occur during or after skin contact with animal(s)? **(#78)** Specify type of animal: _____

- Does H/S occur during or after skin contact with latex material? **(#79)** Specify type of material: _____

- Does H/S occur during or after handling foods? **(#80)** Specify type(s) of food: _____

- Does H/S occur during or after handling drugs? **(#81)** Specify type(s) of drug: _____

- Does H/S occur during or after handling chemicals? **(#82)** Specify type(s) of chemicals: _____

- Does H/S occur during or after contact with cosmetics, shampoo, hair conditioner, soaps, static reducing products for laundry, or detergents? **(#83)** Specify the products: _____

- List any other environmental contacts that may be associated with your symptoms of H/S: _____ _____ _____

N. **Autoimmune disorders (abnormal immune reactions to your own tissues and/or organs). Circle or fill in answers if you develop H/S accompanied by the following symptoms that may be associated with an autoimmune disorder (#84 through #91A):**

- Pain, swelling, tenderness involving joints. **(#84)** Specify symptom: _____ Location:_____

- Dryness of mouth and/or eyes **(#85)**

- Lung symptoms, such as cough, shortness of breath, wheezing **(#86)** Specify symptom: _____ Duration: _____

- Gastrointestinal symptoms, such as vomiting, diarrhea, abdominal cramps, blood in stools **(#87)** Specify symptom:_____ Duration:_____

- Kidney-urinary symptoms, such as reduced frequency of urination, blood in urine, high blood pressure **(#88).** Specify symptom: _____
  Duration:_____

- Muscle symptoms, such as tenderness, pain, or weakness in muscles **(#89)**
  Specify symptom: _____
  Duration:_____ Location:_____

- Skin symptoms, such as sensitivity to sunlight, bruising easily, or the existence of a skin rash other than H/S **(#90).**
  Specify symptom: _____
  Duration:_____ Location:_____

- Thyroid symptoms, such as hair loss, cold intolerance, weight gain, dry skin, lumps or swelling of the thyroid gland (located in front of neck below Adam's apple) **(#91)**

- Swelling with no apparent cause **(#91A)**

- Circle the autoimmune conditions you have:
  Rheumatoid arthritis **(#84, #90)**
  Lupus erythematosus **(#84, #86, #88, #90)**
  Sjogren's syndrome **(#85, #86)**
  Ulcerative colitis, Crohn's disease **(#87, #84)**
  Dermatomyositis **(#89, #90)**
  Autoimmune (Hashimoto's) thyroiditis **(#91)**
  List any other diagnosed autoimmune disease:

  _____

O. Systemic, allergic reaction (anaphylaxis). (# 92)

- Circle any of the following systemic symptoms you have experienced with H/S:
  - Dizziness
  - Loss of consciousness (fainting spells)
  - Low blood pressure

- Metallic taste in your mouth
- Rapid heart rate
- Hoarseness
- Difficulty swallowing
- Sweating
- Itching of palms or soles
- Pale or bluish skin color
- Shortness of breath, rapid breathing rate
- Abdominal cramps, diarrhea or vomiting
- Seizures

- During an episode of H/S, have you:
  - Been on a ventilator
  - Been intubated, (had a breathing tube placed in your windpipe)
  - Had a tracheostomy, (an opening made in your windpipe)

P. Sexual intercourse. Answer these questions if H/S occur during sexual intercourse. (#93)

- Have you experienced H/S during or up to 8 hours after intercourse?

  Yes   No

- If the answer is yes to previous question, have you experienced any of the symptoms of anaphylaxis (see **"O"** section**)** during or up to 8 hours after intercourse?

  Yes   No

  If yes, please describe the symptom(s):

  _____

  _____

  _____

  _____

Q. Record all surgical operation(s) within two years prior to the onset of H/S, (#94).

- ■ Specify the type of surgery and the date:

_____

_____

_____

When you have completed the questionnaire, take it with you to your healthcare professional. Remember to take the photographs and all of your medications and healthcare products. Copies of medication and healthcare product labels are acceptable substitutes if medications are not available.

SECTION 3:

FOR HEALTHCARE
PROFESSIONALS
(HCPs)

INSTRUCTIONS FOR USE OF SECTION 3

"Hives (urticaria) and/or swellings (angioedema)" are frequently abbreviated as H/S in this section.

1. Perform a complete physical examination to confirm the diagnosis of hives and/or swelling. A review of clinical criteria to diagnose these conditions is available in **chapter 2**. **Appendix 1** contains a discussion of the differential diagnoses of these conditions.

2. Review the patient's workbook exercises #1 and#2 (**chapter 3**).
    A. **Exercise 1**:
        Review the photographs to assess the severity of symptoms and confirm that skin lesions are hives and/or swelling.
    B. **Exercise 2**:
        (1) Review the photographs to determine whether skin lesions have disappeared over a 24- to 36-hour interval. If they have not disappeared within 24 to 36 hours, it is possible the skin lesions are not urticaria. Refer to **Appendix 1** to consider the differential diagnosis of hives, such as urticarial vasculitis.
        (2) Review the photographs to determine whether swelling has disappeared within a 24- to 72-hour interval. The HCP should consider other causes in **Appendix 1,** if the swelling does not improve within 72 hours.

3. Review the completed history questionnaire in **chapter 4**. Each symptom or item that has been identified by the patient in the questionnaire (chapter 4) is followed by a bold number. Refer to the same number(s) in **chapter 5** for a discussion of diagnostic possibilities that may be causing these symptoms or conditions and the recommendations for laboratory workup.

4. **Chapter 6** contains general treatment recommendations for H/S. Refer to the same number(s) used in chapters 4 and 5 for recommended treatments for specific diagnosed conditions.

5. The decision to accept the diagnostic suggestions and treatment recommendations should be based on the HCP's integration of the information from the exercises in the workbook, history questionnaire, and physical examination. **This book is not intended to replace the medical judgment of the HCP, who must consider potential clinical benefits versus cost issues when ordering text suggested diagnostic tests**. It should be considered a resource and guide that may assist in the diagnosis and treatment of these conditions.

6. Some discussions and commentary are repeated in this section. Different symptoms can be manifestations of the same disease process. For example, puffiness around the eyes, dry skin, and fatigue may be caused by hypothyroidism secondary to autoimmune thyroiditis. Consequently, several discussions and laboratory recommendations appear more than once in this section.

7. The HCP might consider using **Appendix 3** to record and summarize the evaluation and treatment of patients with H/S.

CHAPTER 5

DIAGNOSTIC CONSIDERATIONS

Each symptom or item that has been identified by the patient in the history questionnaire (chapter 4) is followed by a bold number. Discussions of possible causes of hives and/or swelling for symptoms or items in chapter 4 may be found in chapter 5 by referring to the same number(s). Recommendations for laboratory tests follow each discussion. The healthcare professional should determine the need for these tests based on integration of the workbook information, the questionnaire and the physical examination.

A reference section with supporting citations is located at the end of the book. For example, if you are seeking a reference on exercise-induced anaphylaxis, refer to #33 in the reference section. On occasion, an important citation is noted in the text.

GENERAL ITEMS FROM THE HISTORY QUESTIONNAIRE

#1. HIVES, SWELLING, OR BOTH: CHAPTER 2 AND APPENDIX 1 discuss the criteria for establishing the diagnosis of H/S. If there are no specific leads from the workbook, questionnaire, and diaries (**Appendix 2**), see **chapter 7**. The initial workup for H/S might include screening tests to detect an occult etiology.

RECOMMENDATIONS:

The following screening tests might be considered: CBC, ESR, chemistry profile, ANA profile. Other tests might be considered to rule out unrecognized conditions such as:

- **Autoimmune thyroiditis, (# 54, #55, chapter 5)** may be an occult cause of H/S. A thyroid screen (free T_4, TSH, and perioxidase/thyroglobulin anti-thyroid antibodies) might be appropriate. Positive anti-thyroid antibodies may suggest the presence of autoimmune thyroiditis, which can be associated with H/S. This may occur with hypothyroid, hyperthyroid and euthyroid states.

- **Hereditary and acquired angioedema (#39 for hereditary, and #76 for acquired, chapter 5)** should be considered if unexplained angioedema occurs without hives. A C_4 test would be the minimal screening test, and if the level is decreased, further complement testing is appropriate.

- **Circulating autoantibodies** to IgE or IgE receptors on the surface of mast cells (**chapter 1**) can be assessed by the following method: A small volume (0.05ml) of serum from the patient is injected intradermally into the same individual. A control, consisting of the same volume (0.05 ml) of normal saline, is also injected intradermally. An immediate (10-30 minutes) wheal and flare response with a negative control suggests the presence of circulating autoantibodies. Antihistamines can suppress this response so patients must not take these medications for at least four days prior to the test. Confirmation tests using histamine release and in-vitro methods to detect the presence of circulating autoantibodies exist, but are not available commercially.

The presence of circulating autoantibodies correlates with more severe urticaria compared to chronic urticaria without such autoantibodies. The demonstration of circulating autoantibodies may be useful as a therapeutic marker to justify use of steroids to treat the inflammation of chronic urticaria. In addition, immuno-suppressants, such as cyclophosphamide and cyclosporine (described in **chapter 7**), can decrease the levels of circulating autoantibodies in these patients. Hence, demonstration of circulating autoantibodies may help justify use of these medications in chronic urticaria that is predictably more severe.

- **Urticarial vasculitis (Appendix 1)**. A skin biopsy might be considered to rule out other conditions, such as this masquerader of urticaria.

#2. ACUTE OR CHRONIC SYMPTOMS: Symptoms lasting six weeks or less are considered acute. They are classified as chronic if they are present more than six weeks, either continuously or intermittently.

#3. DAILY PATTERN: The daytime or nighttime pattern is sometimes helpful in making a diagnosis. For example, a nighttime pattern may suggest skin pressure-induced H/S caused by rubbing or scratching during sleep (**# 29, chapter 5**). A daytime pattern could suggest numerous possibilities, such as sunlight-induced H/S (**# 31, chapter 5**).

#4. CONTINUOUS OR INTERMITTENT SYMPTOMS: Knowing whether symptoms are continuous or intermittent may be important. Continuous symptoms may suggest the presence of an underlying medical condition, such as autoimmune thyroiditis. Recurring attacks of hives and/or swelling can have many causes, but one should look for an external trigger, such as exposure to cold temperature or sunlight, relationship to menstrual cycle, or exercise. There are also examples of episodic hives and/or swelling that have no discernible external trigger, such as the syndrome of episodic angioedema associated with eosinophilia (**# 10, chapter 5**).

#5. INITIAL LOCATION OF SYMPTOMS: Knowing what part of the body is first affected with H/S may be helpful in making a diagnosis. For example, a rash that initially involves the head, hands, and feet may not be hives, but rather, a closely-related condition called **erythema multiforme (Appendix 1)**. Classic urticaria usually occurs initially on central body parts such as the chest, abdomen, upper legs and upper arms. Hives that occur on pressure sites, such as soles of feet, buttocks, waist, or under bra straps may suggest dermographism (**# 29, chapter 5**) or deep pressure urticaria (**# 30, chapter 5**).

#6. SEASONAL OCCURRENCE: Seasonality may suggest certain causes. One example is cold-induced urticaria occurring during exposure to a cold environment (**# 32, chapter 5**). Solar urticaria (**# 51, chapter 5**) is triggered by significant sun exposure which occurs more frequently during warmer seasons.

#7. SEVERITY OF SYMPTOMS: The answer to this question assists in knowing whether symptoms are worsening, which would warrant more intensive evaluation and treatment efforts.

The presence of circulating autoantibodies correlates with more severe urticaria compared to chronic urticaria without such autoantibodies. Hence, testing for circulating autoantibodies (**#1, chapter 5**) may be useful in predicting severity of chronic urticaria.

SYMPTOMS OR CONDITIONS

#8. FATIGUE: This common symptom has no specific diagnostic specificity for H/S. It should not be ignored if it persists for several weeks or longer because it may indicate the presence of an underlying systemic disorder that also causes H/S. Fatigue can be associated with many causes of H/S, such as **infections (#58), tumors (#76), autoimmune disorders (#84), hypothyroidism with autoimmune thyroiditis (#54)** and other medical conditions.

RECOMMENDATIONS:
CBC, ESR, mono test, chemistry screen, and a thyroid screen (free T_4, TSH, perioxidase/thyroglobulin anti-thyroid antibodies). Positive anti-thyroid antibodies may suggest the presence of **autoimmune thyroiditis (#54, #55, chapter 5)** accompanied by H/S.

#9. FEVER: Etiologies of this symptom are multiple. The presence of fever may suggest co-existence of an **infectious disease** process. Acute viral illnesses can be associated with the onset of H/S. One particularly interesting association is acute infectious mononucleosis which may induce acquired cold urticaria (**# 32, chapter 5**). Fever is a non-specific symptom. It may be associated with non-infectious inflammatory disease processes, such as **autoimmune diseases** (rheumatoid arthritis, lupus erythematosus). A history suggestive of exposure to viral hepatitis or treatment with penicillin or sulfa drugs, and findings of lymphadenopathy, fever, liver or spleen enlargement upon physical examination, could suggest **serum sickness** as a cause of H/S. Any of these conditions could cause H/S by activating complement (**chapter 1**). The presence of fever excludes allergy as a cause of H/S, since allergy, defined in terms of an immediate IgE antibody-mediated sensitivity to an allergen, is not typically associated with fever. Refer to (**#58A, chapter 5**) for more discussion.

Rare forms of hives and/or swelling associated with fever include: (1) **episodic angioedema with eosinophilia**, urticaria, unexplained weight gain, fever, leukocytosis and elevations of IgM and IgG (**#10, chapter 5**); (2) **Schnitzler's syndrome**, with fever, hives, IgM gammopathy (**#23A, chapter 5**); and (3) familial disorders, such as **Muckle-Wells syndrome** with deafness, nephrosis, hives and fever (**#40, chapter 5**); and **familial auto-inflammatory cold syndrome** with cold-induced fever and a rash that mimics hives (**#32, chapter 5**).

RECOMMENDATIONS:

CBC, ESR, mono test, ANA panel, total complement CH_{50}, appropriate cultures and chemistry screen. A decrease in the level of total complement could suggest several diagnostic possibilities, such as occult infections, and immune complex mediation of serum sickness or systemic autoimmune disease. Circulating immune complex assays (Raji equivalent C_{3D} assay and solid C_{1q} assay) might be considered, if the CH_{50} level is decreased. Other tests depend on the conditions under consideration.

Complement tests require the serum or EDTA plasma specimen be kept on dry ice during transportation.

#10. WEIGHT GAIN: Unexplained weight gain has no diagnostic specificity as a cause of H/S. There are many medical causes of unexplained weight gain such as heart failure, liver disease, renal failure, and capillary leak syndrome.

Unexplained weight gain with H/S could be a manifestation of **hypothyroidism with autoimmune thyroiditis, (# 54, #55, chapter 5)**.

Episodic angioedema with eosinophilia, a rare disorder, has been described with unexplained weight gain (up to 18%). Other symptoms of this syndrome include fever, hives, elevated IgM, and leukocytosis (Gleich et al, 1984).

RECOMMENDATIONS:
CBC, ESR, chemistry screen, thyroid screen (free T_4, TSH, and perioxidase/thyroglobulin anti-thyroid antibodies).

#11. WEIGHT LOSS: Unexplained weight loss has no diagnostic specificity for H/S. Any number of causes could be considered, such as metabolic, malignant, autoimmune, or infectious. Unexplained weight loss with H/S could be a manifestation of **hyperthyroidism associated with autoimmune thyroiditis, (# 54, #55 chapter 5)**.

RECOMMENDATIONS:
CBC, ESR, chemistry screen, ANA profile, and thyroid screen (free T_4, TSH, and perioxidase/thyroglobulin anti-thyroid antibodies).

#12. EMOTIONAL SYMPTOMS: Anxiety reactions, depression, mood swings, and panic may be caused by multiple factors and their concurrence with H/S is often coincidental. However, when these symptoms occur continuously with H/S, they could be a manifestation of a systemic medical disorder that deserves further attention.

Some patients develop rare and unusual appearing hives during stress, referred to as **adrenergic urticaria**. In this condition, typical erythema that surrounds a welt is replaced by a white blanched halo. The cause of this condition is not understood; however there is speculation these patients may have an overactive sympathetic nervous system with increased secretion of adrenalin and noradrenalin.

Another type of hives associated with stress and increased body heat production is **cholinergic urticaria** (**#33, chapter 5**). Patients typically develop pinpoint, itchy hives when they are stressed or overheated during exercise. This condition may reflect an increased sensitivity to acetylcholine released by parasympathetic nerve endings.

Panic and anxiety reactions could be caused by hyperthyroidism with autoimmune thyroiditis **(#55)**.

RECOMMENDATIONS:

CBC, ESR, chemistry screen, thyroid screen (free T_4, TSH, and perioxidase/thyroglobulin anti-thyroid antibodies).

- The diagnosis of **adrenergic urticaria** is made by physical examination, which reveals white halos surrounding wheals.

- A skin test to an acetylcholine derivative, namely Mecholyl® is advised if **cholinergic urticaria** is suspected. The diagnosis of cholinergic urticaria is confirmed if the skin test is positive with wheal and erythema formation in combination with a negative saline control. The Mecholyl® challenge may be positive in only 30% of tested patients with cholinergic urticaria. It may be useful to observe the rash if patients can provoke symptoms during stressful situations. Having patients run on a treadmill in warm clothing or in an occlusive training suit may also provoke symptoms. On rare occasions, some patients with cholinergic urticaria can exhibit symptoms of anaphylaxis. Hence, exercise challenges should be closely monitored.

#13. DRY SKIN: Dry skin has no diagnostic specificity for H/S. However, dry skin can cause itching, which could exacerbate conditions, such as dermographism (**# 29, chapter 5**). Dry skin with H/S could also be a manifestation of **hypothyroidism with autoimmune thyroiditis, (# 54, chapter 5)**.

RECOMMENDATIONS:

CBC, chemistry screen, test for dermographism (**# 29, chapter 5**), thyroid screen (free T_4, TSH, and perioxidase/thyroglobulin anti-thyroid antibodies).

#14. BRUISING EASILY: Easy bruising tendency has no diagnostic specificity for H/S. However, several possibilities should be considered as a cause of H/S, such as (1) **urticarial vasculitis (Appendix 1)**; (2) blood disorders (**chronic lymphocytic leukemia**); (3) autoimmune disorders (lupus erythematosus); and (4) the effect of long-term **steroid therapy**.

RECOMMENDATIONS:

CBC, platelet count, ESR, bleeding time and possibly a coagulation workup, chemistry screen, total complement CH_{50}, ANA profile, and a skin biopsy.

Complement tests require the serum or EDTA plasma specimen be kept on dry ice during transportation.

#15. HAIR LOSS: Hair loss has no diagnostic specificity as it may occur with systemic diseases such as lupus erythematosus, or following surgery and febrile illnesses. However, hair loss occurring with H/S could be a manifestation of **hypothyroidism with autoimmune thyroiditis (#54, chapter 5)**.

RECOMMENDATIONS:

CBC, ESR, ANA panel, chemistry screen, thyroid screen (free T_4, TSH, and perioxidase/thyroglobulin anti-thyroid antibodies).

#16, #17, #21. TENDERNESS OVER FACE; DISCOLORED NASAL DISCHARGE; PAINFUL TEETH: These symptoms have no diagnostic specificity for H/S. However, they could be a manifestation of an underlying disorder such as a **sinus infection (#64, chapter 5)**. Tenderness over the face and teeth may also suggest a **tooth abscess or gingivitis**. The existence of an occult infection could cause H/S by activating complement (**chapter 1 and "history of recent infection" #58, chapter 5**).

RECOMMENDATIONS:

CBC, ESR, total complement CH_{50}, X-ray or preferably a CT scan of sinuses. Dental X-rays may also be advised.

Complement tests require the serum or EDTA plasma specimen be kept on dry ice during transportation.

#18. PUFFINESS AROUND EYES: Periocular puffiness has no diagnostic specificity for H/S. There are many causes of unexplained periocular puffiness, such as fluid retention from heart, liver, or kidney disease, or inflammation from an autoimmune disease (i.e. dermatomyositis). This symptom could be a manifestation of underlying disorders associated with H/S, such as **hypothyroidism from autoimmune thyroiditis, (# 54, chapter 5)** or **contact allergic dermatitis (#77)**.

RECOMMENDATIONS:

- CBC, ESR, chemistry screen for routine workup. ANA and ENA panels if an **autoimmune disorder** is suspected.

- If there is a suspicion of **hypothyroidism from autoimmune thyroiditis**, include free T_4, TSH, and perioxidase/thyroglobulin anti-thyroid antibodies.

- Other considerations might be **contact allergic sensitivity** to facial skin products including shampoos and hair conditioners with foreign animal proteins and/or nettle. Removal of all facial skin products for one week would be recommended.

- Contact patch testing to facial products should be considered. Diluted topical products should be applied onto aluminum discs (Finn Chambers) when performing patch tests. The chambers can be purchased at Allerderm Company, Petaluma CA, (www.allerderm.com). It is advisable to dilute chemicals and products before patch testing to avoid severe irritant reactions. Allerderm can provide information on appropriate dilutions for testing common topical products. A good reference for proper patch test dilution is listed in the reference section (DeGroot AC, 1994). Common patch test chemicals and allergens can be ordered from Allerderm (Petaluma, CA) for use with T.R.U.E. test kits. More unusual patch test chemicals can be ordered from Pharmascience Inc. (Montreal, Canada). A dermatologist or allergist can also provide guidance. Patch tests to these materials should be read 30 minutes after application and again at 48 and 72 hours.

#19. SEVERE SORE THROAT; DIFFICULTY SWALLOWING; RECURRING HOARSENESS:
These symptoms have many causes and no diagnostic specificity for H/S. Sore throat occurring with H/S could be a manifestation of **infectious mononucleosis, strepto-coccal infection, postnasal drainage from sinusitis or caused by other infectious diseases**. An occult infection could cause H/S by activating complement (**chapter 1 and discussion "history of recent infection" #58, chapter 5**).

Recurring **hoarseness and difficulty swallowing** can be a manifestation of angioedema. Both symptoms are considered life-threatening because they may signify swelling within or around the vocal cords. This region is very susceptible to swelling because of the high concentration of mast cells in the larynx and vocal cord area. The cause of swelling in this region is multiple and can include: **food sensitivity (#52, chapter 5); drug sensitivity (# 50, chapter 5); inhalant sensitivity (#33, chapter 5); hereditary and acquired angioedema (#39 for hereditary and #76 for acquired angioedema, chapter 5); insect sensitivity reactions (# 51, chapter 5); exercise induced H/S (# 33, chapter 5).**

RECOMMENDATIONS:

- For **sore throat and sinusitis**: CBC, ESR, throat culture, streptozyme test, mono test and possibly total complement CH_{50}. Complement tests require the serum or EDTA plasma specimen be kept on dry ice when transported. Evaluation for sinusitis may include sinus X-rays or CT screening of sinuses.

- For **hoarseness and difficult swallowing**: CBC, ESR, and appropriate skin tests, or IgE RAST blood tests may be indicated for sensitivity to inhalants, foods, insect venoms or drugs. An exercise challenge test should be ordered if the history is appropriate, and performed under medical supervision. Nasal-laryngeal fiberoscopy may be necessary to determine the location of swelling.

- Total complement CH_{50}, C_4, and C_{1q} might be indicated. A decreased C_4 level warrants quantitative and functional C_1 esterase inhibitor assays. A decrease in levels of either assay may indicate a hereditary disorder. The pattern of inheritance for hereditary angioedema is autosomal co-dominant, but occurrence in a single generation due to spontaneous mutation has been reported.

A decreased C_{1q} suggests further evaluation to rule out acquired angioedema, possibly due to a lymphoproliferative malignancy, or an autoimmune disorder associated with an autoantibody to C_1 esterase inhibitor. Recent studies indicate patients with autoantibodies to C_1 esterase inhibitor may eventually develop a malignant lymphoproliferative disorder. Continued surveillance for this possibility is advised. A neoplasm evaluation might include immunotyping of peripheral blood lymphocytes for the detection of malignant B cells; serum protein immunoelectrophoresis and immunofixation to rule out dysproteinemia; T and B cell gene rearrangement with PCR amplification to detect occult T and/or B cell neoplasms; and CT of the chest, abdomen, and pelvis to rule out a lymphoma or other neoplasm.

Complement tests require the serum or EDTA plasma specimen be kept on dry ice during transportation.

#20. COLD SORES: Recurring cold sores are frequently caused by viral infections, especially by Herpes Simplex virus. Chronic **Herpes Simplex infections** have been associated with a skin disorder that can masquerade as urticaria, i.e. **erythema multiforme (Appendix 1)**.

RECOMMENDATIONS:
CBC, ESR, Herpes Simplex virus antibody titer (obtain baseline serum and a serum specimen three to four weeks later to determine whether there has been a rise in the titer of this antibody).

#21. TEETH ARE PAINFUL: (see #16, #17, chapter 5).

#22, #23. JOINT PAIN; JOINT SWELLING: Causes are multiple and have no diagnostic specificity for H/S. However joint symptoms that occur in combination with H/S could be manifestations of a systemic disease, such as an **autoimmune disorder (chapter 1)**, **systemic vasculitis** with **urticarial vasculitis (Appendix 1) or serum sickness**.

RECOMMENDATIONS:

CBC, ESR, chemistry screen, total complement CH_{50}, ANA profile, rheumatoid factor, skin biopsy, and appropriate X-rays of joints.

Complement tests require the serum or EDTA plasma specimen be kept on dry ice during transportation.

#23A. BONE PAIN: The association of bone pain with H/S has no diagnostic specificity. Diagnostic considerations might include **systemic mastocytosis**. The former is associated with overproduction of mast cells in the bone marrow (**# 29, chapter 5**). A rare form of non-pruritic chronic hives with bone pain is **Schnitzler's syndrome,** a disorder characterized by monoclonal IgM, anemia, fever, fatigue and weight loss. Other gammopathies associated with bone pain have been associated with hives.

RECOMMENDATIONS:

CBC, ESR, chemistry screen, ANA profile, alpha tryptase for mastocytosis, serum immunofixation to detect monoclonal peaks, skin biopsy, possibly a bone marrow biopsy and appropriate bone X-rays.

#24. MULTIPLE BONE FRACTURES: H/S can be associated with **hyperparathyroidism** which may cause multiple bone fractures. An overactive parathyroid can induce calcium release from bones. It is thought that H/S is caused by calcium induced mediator (histamine) release from mast cells.

RECOMMENDATIONS:

CBC, ESR, total calcium, ionized calcium, parathyroid hormone and parathyroid hormone-related protein (PTHrP).

#25. CHRONIC COUGH, SHORTNESS OF BREATH, WHEEZING: There is some literature describing lung diseases in combination with H/S in which the lung disease is considered the cause of H/S or the manifestation of a systemic disease with H/S. Lung disorders that have been described with H/S include **cancer of the lung, autoimmune disease, and systemic vasculitis**. Wheezing that accompanies H/S may suggest an anaphylactic event. No mechanism is known to explain the sporadic occurrence of H/S with lung cancer.

RECOMMENDATIONS:
CBC, ESR, ANA profile, chemistry screen, chest X-ray, and pulmonary function tests. An elevated serum beta tryptase would provide evidence that wheezing with H/S is associated with an anaphylactic event. This test must be ordered within **two hours** of the onset of wheezing to detect an elevated level.

#26. GASTROINTESTINAL SYMPTOMS: Some literature describes the association of gastrointestinal (GI) diseases with H/S, where either the GI disease is considered to be the cause of H/S, or a manifestation of a systemic disease that includes H/S.

GENERAL RECOMMENDATIONS:
CBC, ESR, and chemistry screen.

#26A. INFLAMMATORY BOWEL DISEASE may present with abdominal pains, fever, loss of weight and blood in stools. No mechanism is known to explain the sporadic occurrence of inflammatory bowel disease and H/S, although both may be manifestations of a systemic autoimmune disorder. Another theory suggests inflammatory bowel disease may be associated with increased permeability of the intestine, allowing large immunogenic food molecules to be absorbed. These food antigens may cause abnormal immune responses, such as immune complex formation or IgE antibody responses.

RECOMMENDATIONS:
GI X-rays, endoscopy and referral to a gastroenterologist may be required.

#26B. CELIAC DISEASE may present with fatigue, diarrhea, weight loss (despite normal caloric intake), and intolerance to grains containing gluten, which may cause abdominal cramps. No mechanism is known to explain the sporadic occurrence of H/S and celiac disease, although both may be manifestations of a systemic autoimmune disorder. Another theory suggests celiac disease may be associated with increased permeability of the intestine, allowing large immunogenic food molecules to be absorbed. These food antigens may cause abnormal immune responses, such as immune complex formation or IgE antibody responses.

RECOMMENDATIONS:

Gluten antibody blood tests (Gliadin IgG, Gliadin IgA), transglutaminase, GI X-rays, endoscopy, and referral to a gastroenterologist for potential bowel biopsy. A therapeutic trial with a gluten-free diet may be helpful in making the diagnosis.

#26C. PARASITIC DISEASE may be characterized by watery, sometimes bloody

stools. The *Giardia lamblia* parasite is probably the most common parasite acquired in the U.S and has been reported to cause H/S. It is transmitted by ingesting water contaminated by *Giardia* in deer and animal feces. *Giardia* can be acquired by drinking contaminated water from a well, river, pond, lake, and other unpurified water sources. No mechanism is known to explain the occurrence of H/S with parasitic infections, although it is tempting to consider that H/S is caused by an immune response to parasites, such as by the activation of complement (**chapter 1 and "history of recent infection" #58, chapter 5**), or by an immediate IgE antibody-mediated sensitivity to a parasitic allergen (**chapter 1**).

RECOMMENDATIONS:

Ova and parasite stool examination on several specimens, and if appropriate, referral to a gastroenterologist to obtain duodenal aspirates to rule out *Giardia* infestation. IgE levels are sometimes elevated.

#26D. VIRAL HEPATITIS symptoms may include fatigue, fever, dark urine, light-col-

ored stools, jaundice and tenderness over the right upper quadrant of the abdomen. Certain individuals may be at high risk for hepatitis, such as, medical personnel with a history of needle-sticks or exposure to body fluids, persons who have recently traveled to foreign countries (especially third world nations), the use of illegal intravenous drugs, and persons who have received blood transfusions. The occurrence of H/S with viral hepatitis is thought to be the result of immune complex formation and complement activation (**chapter 1**).

RECOMMENDATIONS:

Profiles for hepatitis types A, B, and C would be indicated, total complement CH_{50}, and a skin biopsy may also be ordered if urticarial vasculitis accompanies the hepatitis (**Appendix 1**). A referral to a gastroenterologist would be indicated if the diagnosis is confirmed.

Complement tests require the serum or EDTA plasma specimen be kept on dry ice during transportation.

#26E. HEREDITARY OR ACQUIRED ANGIOEDEMA may induce swelling of the gastrointestinal tract and cause abdominal cramps and pain. **Urticaria is not associated with this condition**. Hereditary angioedema is a potentially fatal disease, especially if swelling affects the upper airway. However, it can be diagnosed easily and treated effectively. A quantitative deficiency in C_1 esterase inhibitor is observed in most cases of hereditary angioedema (**#39, chapter 5**). Some patients with hereditary angioedema (15%) have normal quantitative levels of C_1 esterase inhibitor with an abnormal functional assay of C_1 esterase inhibitor. Patients with hereditary angioedema exhibit an autosomal dominant pattern of inheritance, but there are isolated cases that have occurred in a single generation due to spontaneous mutation.

An underlying lymphoma, other cancers, infectious diseases (hepatitis B, HIV), or an autoimmune disease should be considered, if the C_{1q} level is decreased.

RECOMMENDATIONS:

The evaluation to rule out gastrointestinal swelling caused by **hereditary or acquired angioedema** would include C_4, quantitative and functional assays for C_1 esterase inhibitor, and C_{1q}. A decrease in the C_4 level or quantitative/functional assays for C_1 esterase inhibitor should prompt referral to an allergist or immunologist. Complement tests require the serum or EDTA plasma specimen be kept on dry ice during transportation.

A decreased C_{1q} level may necessitate an evaluation for an occult lymphoma or other conditions (**#39, chapter 5**). Antibody to C_1 esterase inhibitor may be positive if an acquired autoimmune disorder is considered. An ANA profile would also be indicated. Recent studies indicate patients with autoantibody to C_1 esterase inhibitor may eventually develop a malignant lymphoproliferative disorder. Continued surveillance for this possibility is advised. A neoplasm evaluation might include immunotyping of peripheral blood lymphocytes for the detection of malignant B cells; serum protein immunoelectrophoresis and immunofixation to rule out dysproteinemia; T and B cell gene rearrangement with PCR amplification to detect an occult T and/or B cell neoplasm; and CT of the chest, abdomen, and pelvis to rule out a lymphoma or other neoplasm. Both acquired and hereditary angioedema may exhibit a pattern of "picket fence" edema on GI X-rays.

#26F. ULCERS OF THE STOMACH AND DUODENUM can be caused by an underlying bacterial infection (*Helicobacter pylori*). Some investigators have suggested that H. *pylori* can also cause H/S. However this cause-effect relationship remains controversial. The presence of "heart burn", reflux of stomach acids into the mouth and larynx sometimes associated with cough, abdominal pain, vomiting, and dark black stools, may be suggestive of gastrointestinal ulcers. No mechanism is known to explain the occurrence of H/S with H. *pylori* infections, although the theory of molecular mimicry has been proposed. This concept would suggest H. *pylori* stimulates the production of antibodies with homology to IgE or IgE receptors, which in turn are capable of inducing hives and/or swelling.

RECOMMENDATIONS:

The association of H/S with **ulcers** may indicate the need for a referral to a gastroenterologist to rule out the co-existence of *Helicobacter pylori* infection. Tests may include an IgG antibody blood test for H. *pylori*, C urea breath test and upper gastrointestinal endoscopy.

#27. SYMPTOMS INVOLVING URINARY AND/OR REPRODUCTIVE SYSTEMS: Urinary and/or reproductive system disease has been described in the medical literature as a cause of H/S, or a manifestation of a systemic disease that includes H/S. The urinary and reproductive disorders listed below are sometimes associated with H/S:

GENERAL RECOMMENDATIONS:
CBC, ESR, chemistry screen, and urinalysis.

#27A, #27B, #27D. TESTICULAR CANCER; OVARIAN CANCER; KIDNEY CANCER.

The mechanism causing the concurrence of H/S with these cancers has not been identified, although one theory is that cancer-induced circulating immune complexes might be responsible.

RECOMMENDATIONS:

The diagnosis is established primarily by physical examination and radiological studies. Referral would be appropriate if a diagnosis is confirmed or suspected. Ordering an evaluation for immune complex mediation might be useful in understanding the mechanism, such as total complement (CH_{50}) and immune complex assays (Raji equivalent C_{3D} assay and solid C_{1q} assay). Complement tests require the serum or EDTA plasma specimen be kept on dry ice during transportation.

#27C. GLOMERULONEPHRITIS AND URTICARIAL VASCULITIS (APPENDIX 1); NEPHROTIC SYNDROME.

Glomerulonephritis and urticarial vasculitis can be manifestations of systemic vasculitis mediated by immune complexes.

Muckle-Wells syndrome **(#40, chapter 5)** is an autosomal dominant syndrome characterized by chronic nephrosis due to AA amyloidosis, occasional deafness, periodic fever and urticaria. It is caused by mutations on the same gene associated with Familial Cold Auto-inflammatory syndrome **(#32, chapter 5)**. Interleukin-1 is thought to be involved as it contributes to increased synthesis of serum amyloid A.

RECOMMENDATIONS:

Screening tests may include urinalysis, BUN, and creatinine clearance. Referral to a nephrologist may be necessary. A skin biopsy and total complement CH_{50} would be appropriate to rule out urticarial vasculitis.

Ordering an evaluation for immune complex mediation could be useful in understanding the mechanism, such as immune complex assays (Raji equivalent C_{3D} assay and solid C_{1q} assay). Complement tests require the serum or EDTA plasma specimen be kept on dry ice during transportation.

Diagnostic genotype for Muckle-Wells syndrome can be obtained by contacting Hal Hoffman, M.D. (hahoffman@ucsd.edu).

#27E. INTERSTITIAL CYSTITIS. No mechanism is known to explain the sporadic occurrence of H/S with this bladder disease. Interstitial cystitis causes painful, frequent urination without evidence of an active infection.

RECOMMENDATIONS:
Evaluation may require urine culture and cystoscopy by a urologist.

#27F. SEXUALLY TRANSMITTED DISEASES: Several sexually transmitted diseases have been associated with H/S, such as syphilis, gonorrhea, trichomonas, and HIV. It is speculated infectious diseases could cause H/S by activating complement, (**chapter 1 and "history of recent infection" #58, chapter 5**).

RECOMMENDATIONS:
The following tests would be appropriate, depending on the history and physical examination: syphilis serology, culture of genital secretions, microscopic examination of genital secretions, and an HIV test.

Ordering an evaluation for immune complex mediation, such as total complement CH_{50} and immune complex assays (Raji equivalent C_{3D} assay and solid C_{1q} assay), could be useful in understanding the mechanism. Complement tests require the serum or EDTA plasma specimen be kept on dry ice during transportation.

#27G. H/S COINCIDING WITH MENSTRUAL CYCLES. This syndrome may be caused by allergic IgE antibody sensitivity to endogenous progesterone.

RECOMMENDATIONS:

IgE allergic antibodies to progesterone may be detected by skin testing to aqueous progesterone or its analog, medroxyprogesterone. Skin testing with medroxyprogesterone should be performed cautiously because anaphylaxis has been reported when testing with this compound. The test should be diluted significantly to prevent sloughing of the surrounding skin, (**chapter 5, #57**).

#27H. A SECOND SYNDROME OF H/S COINCIDING WITH MENSTRUAL CYCLES.

Reduced progesterone levels may cause this syndrome.

RECOMMENDATIONS:

Total eosinophil counts and serum progesterone levels are advised. In this rare syndrome, eosinophil counts are elevated and serum progesterone levels are reduced when the patient is symptomatic.

#28. SYMPTOMS OF MUSCLE AND/OR NERVE DISEASE: Muscle or nerve system diseases have been described in the medical literature as a cause of H/S, or a manifestation of a systemic disease that includes H/S.

GENERAL RECOMMENDATIONS:

A detailed muscle and neurological examination. Initial screening tests may include CBC, ESR, chemistry screen, and ANA profile.

#28A. POLYMYOSITIS may cause muscle pain and weakness. No mechanism is known to explain the sporadic association of H/S with this condition.

RECOMMENDATIONS:

Serum creatine kinase and aldolase are advised, as they may be elevated in these conditions. Electromyographic and muscle biopsy abnormalities may be suggestive of the diagnosis. Referral to a neurologist may be indicated.

#28B. GAMMOPATHY may cause neurological symptoms, bone pain, fatigue, pallor, loss of weight and other symptoms. No mechanism is known to explain the sporadic association of H/S with gammopathies, although immune complex formation and complement activation could be involved.

RECOMMENDATIONS:

Serum protein electrophoresis, immunofixation, appropriate bone X-rays, bone marrow examination, and referral to a hematologist or an oncologist would be warranted if gammopathy is suspected or diagnosed.

An evaluation for immune complex mediation could be useful in understanding the mechanism causing H/S in association with a gammopathy. Appropriate tests would be total complement CH_{50} and immune complex assays (Raji equivalent C_{3D} assay and solid C_{1q} assay). Complement tests require the serum or EDTA plasma specimen be kept on dry ice during transportation.

#28C. HERPES ZOSTER ("shingles") causes a chickenpox-like rash overlying a painful region of skin. No mechanism is known to explain the sporadic association of H/S with this condition.

RECOMMENDATIONS:

The diagnosis is made by physical examination, although specific antibody tests and skin biopsy findings may confirm it.

#28D. SYSTEMIC VASCULITIS that involves muscle and/or neurological systems in combination with urticarial vasculitis (**Appendix 1**). Occasionally angioedema can accompany urticarial vasculitis.

RECOMMENDATIONS:

A skin biopsy may reveal histo-pathological evidence of urticarial vasculitis. Total complement CH_{50} may be normal or decreased. An ANA panel should be included. If this diagnosis is a serious consideration, a referral to a neurologist and/or allergist-clinical immunologist would be appropriate.

An evaluation for immune complex mediation could be useful in understanding the mechanism causing H/S in association with systemic vasculitis. Appropriate tests would be total complement CH_{50} and immune complex assays (Raji equivalent C_{3D} assay and solid C_{1q} assay). Complement tests require the serum or EDTA plasma specimen be kept on dry ice during transportation.

#28E. AUTOIMMUNE DISEASES, such as **dermatomyositis**, may cause weakness in large muscle groups involving the upper legs, upper arms and shoulders, periocular redness with puffiness, and a salmon-colored rash on the knuckles of the hands. Muscle weakness may be noticed when walking upstairs, getting out of a bathtub, or carrying groceries. Dermatomyositis can be associated with underlying malignancies. No mechanism is known to explain the association of H/S with an autoimmune disease, other than speculation that all symptoms are manifestations of a systemic autoimmune disorder.

RECOMMENDATIONS:
ANA profile, skin biopsy, evaluation for underlying visceral malignancy associated with dermatomyositis and referral to a rheumatologist and/or immunologist.

#29. INDUCTION OF URTICARIA BY RUBBING OR SCRATCHING: Patients notice that rubbing or scratching their skin will induce welts (hives). This condition is referred to as **dermographism** or dermatographism. The origin of the word is from "derm" which means skin and "graph" refers to writing, so literally, the word refers to the ability to write on skin. The cause of this condition is unknown, but may develop after a **drug reaction** or from an **infectious illness, usually viral** in nature. There is often no known cause for this condition. It is not generally an inherited disorder, although familial autosomal dominant dermographism has been described in several families **(#36A, chapter 5)**. Affected patients will notice welts on their face, neck or torso after rubbing or scratching their skin, especially during sleep. Welts can also occur on areas constrained by tight garments, such as the waist due to wearing a tight belt, or the lower legs from wearing close-fitting socks. This condition generally improves spontaneously, and is of less concern once patients are aware they can prevent symptoms by not rubbing and scratching their skin and by wearing looser garments. No mechanism is known to explain this condition. One study implicates IgE antibody mediation.

A sub-group of patients exhibit **biphasic dermographism**. After the resolution of the immediate dermographic response, patients develop raised erythematous pruritic lesions 3 to 8 hours later at the same location **(delayed dermographism)**. The late phase is probably due to a cellular inflammatory response, similar to late phase inflammation which occurs in biphasic anaphylaxis.

There are more serious conditions associated with welts induced by scratching or rubbing. These conditions are referred to as **mastocytosis** and **urticaria pigmentosa**. In both conditions there is an overproduction of mast cells in the skin, which release mediators following rubbing or scratching. Mastocytosis is a systemic condition in which mast cells accumulate in internal organs and the skin. Symptoms can include pruritis, flushing, nausea, vomiting, abdominal pain, tachycardia, headaches, and fatigue. In some circumstances the condition can evolve into a malignant disease.

Clusters of mast cells appear as dark brown, freckle-like skin lesions in urticaria pigmentosa and mastocytosis. Rubbing or scratching in a straight line over an affected area of skin may help differentiate normal freckles, dermographism, mastocytosis and urticaria pigmentosa. Rubbing normally-pigmented freckles may produce a red streak that rapidly disappears but does not produce a welt. Rubbing or scratching the pigmented skin lesions of mastocytosis or urticaria pigmentosa will induce welts with varying diameters that are often separated from each other. Rubbing dermographic skin will produce a line of continuous welts with almost equal diameters.

RECOMMENDATIONS:
- CBC, ESR, chemistry screen, and ANA profile.

- Test for **dermographism, mastocytosis and urticaria pigmentosa** by rubbing the skin with the edge of a tongue blade or similar dull instrument. Have the patient check 4 to 8 hours later to determine whether there is a delayed response at the same location, which is characteristic of **delayed dermographism**. More precise testing for dermographism can be done with a dermographometer that applies graded pressure to induce skin responses. An alpha tryptase level and a skin biopsy with Giemsa staining are appropriate tests to confirm the diagnosis of urticaria pigmentosa and mastocytosis. Both conditions reveal increased levels of total tryptase (>20ng/ml) in which alpha tryptase is the predominant type. Serum tryptase can be moderately elevated in chronic idiopathic urticaria (Bruno et al, 2001), and in some cases, the elevation can be caused by unrecognized allergic reactions. Increased numbers of mast cells in skin biopsies are also observed in mastocytosis and urticaria pigmentosa. The selected site for skin biopsy should be a non-traumatized location to allow the detection of intact granules in mast cells. A bone marrow biopsy may be indicated for an evaluation of systemic mastocytosis. A referral to a clinical immunologist, allergist or dermatologist would be appropriate, if the diagnosis of mastocytosis or urticaria pigmentosa is strongly considered or confirmed.

#30. PAINFUL SWELLING FROM SUSTAINED PRESSURE: This condition is called **delayed pressure urticaria** and refers to swelling that appears several hours after an anatomical region is subjected to repetitive or sustained pressure. The term urticaria may be a misnomer for this condition because the swelling of delayed pressure urticaria is diffuse and deep under the skin surface, which is different from the superficial, discrete swelling characteristic of classic urticaria. *In some respects, the swelling of deep pressure urticaria is more angioedema-like and for that reason, a more appropriate name might be deep pressure angioedema.* Typically, deep pressure urticaria develops two to six hours after the applied pressure has been discontinued. The swelling is usually very painful, especially when it involves anatomically confined areas that restrict significant swelling. Examples include:

- Painful swelling of a finger or hand, caused by repetitive use of a tool (e.g. hammer, screwdriver or power tool).

- Painful swelling of the feet, caused by standing for long periods, walking or running.

- Painful swelling of shoulders, arms, or hands after carrying heavy objects.

- Painful swelling of exercised muscle groups, caused by weight-lifting.

The condition is acquired for unknown reasons and is more common in young adult males. Other symptoms may be associated with delayed pressure urticaria, such as low-grade fever, muscle pain, and fatigue. A few medical articles suggest abnormal immune responses to ingested foods may be an underlying cause or trigger of this condition.

Angioedema should be considered in the differential diagnosis, since the swelling of delayed pressure urticaria is diffuse, deep, painful at times, and asymmetrical. **Hereditary and acquired angioedema** should be considered in this discussion, as mild trauma can elicit symptoms in these syndromes.

RECOMMENDATIONS:

- A screening test for **delayed pressure urticaria** is advised. Apply a 10- to 15-pound weight on a shoulder for fifteen minutes. There is usually no immediate swelling after removing the weight; however, diffuse deep swelling may develop at the pressure site two to six hours later. The response is diagnostic of this condition. Pressure tests can sometimes give false negative results for the following reasons:

  - Some areas of the skin are less responsive than others. If the test is negative on the shoulder, a repeat test can be performed on the back.

  - The weights may be too light and should be increased to test for pressure sensitivity.

  - An area that was swollen recently may be refractory to challenge. Pressure testing needs to be performed at a different location.

  - Steroids can suppress the response. Hence, steroids need to be discontinued for a minimum of four days prior to the pressure test.

Other tests include: CBC, ESR, chemistry screen, ANA profile, and allergy skin tests (skin puncture method) to a panel of foods commonly ingested by the affected individual. The skin puncture tests should be read fifteen minutes, and again four to six hours after application. Erythema and swelling at four to six hours are considered positive endpoints and may implicate a food as a cause or trigger of this condition. The ESR may be elevated, suggesting the condition is caused by an inflammatory mechanism.

- Tests for **angioedema** might include: C_4, C_{1q} and CH_{50}. Quantitative and functional C_1 esterase inhibitor assays would be warranted to rule out **hereditary angioedema** if the C_4 level is decreased. This disorder usually occurs with a multi-generational autosomal co-dominant pattern of inheritance, but testing may be warranted without a family history because spontaneous mutations of C_1 esterase inhibitor have been reported (**#39, chapter 5**). An evaluation for **acquired angioedema** would be appropriate if the C_{1q} level is decreased (**#39 and #76, chapter 5**).

#31. EXPOSURE TO SUNLIGHT: This is a rare condition in which urticaria develops following sunlight exposure and is referred to as **solar urticaria.** Typically, a patient will observe hives on areas exposed to sunlight. No mechanism is known to explain this condition, although there is speculation that IgE antibodies are formed against a skin protein which has been altered by sunlight. Additional studies are needed to prove this theory.

A consultation with a dermatologist may be needed to differentiate it from other light or sunlight sensitive skin conditions, such as porphyrias, polymorphic light eruption, drug sensitivity, and lupus erythematosus. In comparison to solar urticaria, most of these sunlight-induced conditions exhibit skin eruptions which take many days to disappear. Additionally, direct skin contact with chemicals, drugs or foods, in combination with light exposure, can induce **contact photo-allergic sensitivity,** which is manifested by hive-like reactions. Perfumes applied to the "V" area of the neck can cause photo-allergic reactions. Handling certain foods, such as raw celery, can also induce contact photo-allergic urticaria.

RECOMMENDATIONS:

- Positive sunlight induction of urticaria is diagnostic of **solar urticaria**. Patients should be advised to avoid using antihistamines or sunscreens, and then expose themselves to the same sunlight conditions that induced symptoms. A dermatologist, using light sources at specific wavelengths, can perform more refined testing. Other recommended tests include: CBC, ESR, chemistry screen, and ANA profile. Referral to an allergist or dermatologist may be appropriate.

- A more detailed history for cosmetics and food handling should be included in the workup to determine if the patient is exposed to a substance that might induce **contact photo-allergic urticaria**. An allergist or dermatologist can perform diagnostic photo-contact patch tests.

#32. COLD EXPOSURE: When a patient describes hives during or after environmental cold exposure, they are sometimes doubted and even questioned about their psychological health. This is a real medical condition in which individuals develop H/S during or after exposure to cold temperatures. The general condition is called **acquired cold urticaria.** The onset of this disorder can be sudden and may occur without warning, such as a person who swims and notices the onset of H/S without a prior history of these symptoms. Under extreme circumstances, individuals with this condition can develop dizziness, low blood pressure and lose consciousness, which may cause drowning. Less dramatic examples include a child who develops swelling of the mouth and lips after eating ice cream or a person developing hives in areas exposed to cold temperature, such as the face during skiing. The diagnosis of acquired cold urticaria can be established by a cold stimulation test that is described in the recommendations of this section.

This condition can be acquired at any age; however, the usual onset occurs in younger age groups. Acquired cold urticaria with no recognized underlying cause is referred to as **primary acquired cold urticaria**. One theory suggests cold-sensitive circulating IgG or IgM autoantibodies to IgE may be responsible for this condition. Another theory has implicated IgE antibodies to an unidentified cold-sensitive skin antigen. Acquired cold urticaria may occasionally occur secondarily to other disorders (**secondary acquired cold urticaria**), such as **infectious mononucleosis, syphilis, HIV, hepatitis C, mycoplasma infections, chronic lymphocytic leukemia, vasculitis and cryoglobulinemia**.

Some patients with convincing histories of cold urticaria cannot be diagnosed with a cold stimulation test. These individuals are diagnosed as having **atypical cold urticaria.** They apparently require a cold temperature warmer than ice to induce symptoms.

There are two inherited cold sensitivity disorders. **Familial cold urticaria** has been renamed **familial cold auto-inflammatory syndrome (#37, chapter 5)**. It is characterized by the onset of fever, chills, a measles-like rash, joint pains, and conjunctivitis, all occurring a few hours after cold exposure. The rash in this condition is **not** urticaria, as it is more measles-like, not itchy, and will remain for more than 24 to 36 hours. The genetic pattern of this condition is autosomal dominant, although spontaneous mutations have been described. A multi-generational family history may not be necessary to consider this diagnosis. The gene producing the abnormal cryopyrin protein that causes this disorder has recently been located on the first chromosome (1q44). Mutations of the same gene cause Muckle-Wells **(#40)**.

The other familial cold disorder is called **delayed cold urticaria (#38, chapter 5)** and is characterized by the development of urticaria several hours after exposure to cold. It is also inherited in an autosomal dominant pattern.

RECOMMENDATIONS:

- A cold stimulation test for **primary and secondary acquired cold urticaria** is advised. Patients who undergo cold testing must not take antihistamines for a minimum of four days prior to the test. A cold object, such as a small plastic bag filled with ice, is applied to the forearm for five minutes. After removal, the skin should be allowed to re-warm to normal body temperature and then be inspected for wheal development that often has the shape of the test object. The appearance of a wheal is diagnostic of cold urticaria. There are some patients who require longer periods of cold stimulation (10 to 15 minutes) to stimulate a wheal response. Retesting should be performed at different skin locations, since repeat testing on the same skin site will cause localized tolerance to cold temperature.

On occasion, it may be necessary to perform a more detailed cold stimulation test called the **cold stimulation time test (CSTT)**. It measures the minimum time of cold contact required to induce an immediate coalescent wheal. A cold stimulus (ice cube in a plastic bag) is applied to the subject's skin, usually the forearm, at 1 minute intervals up to 10 minutes until a coalescent wheal is induced. For example, a CSTT test might begin at 1 minute. If it is negative, the next CSTT would be 2 minutes etc. until a coalescent wheal is elicited, which represents the minimum time of cold contact for induction of a positive test. Each test is recorded after the skin has re-warmed. During the CSTT the cold stimulus is never applied to the same skin site to avoid testing skin areas which may have become desensitized to cold. The CSTT can be used over time to determine whether patients are improving spontaneously. There is an excellent correlation between resolution of cold urticaria and prolongation of the CSTT result. The same applies when monitoring patients who are taking suppressive antihistamines. Cold sensitivity generally improves if the CSTT is increased while taking an antihistamine.

- Other tests for **secondary acquired cold urticaria** may include: CBC, ESR, chemistry screen, ANA profile, cryoglobulin, cold agglutinins, syphilis serology, HIV, and an infectious mononucleosis test.

The cryoglobulin test must be performed correctly or false negative results can occur. Once the blood is obtained, it should **not** be placed in a refrigerator or packed on ice because the cryoglobulin can precipitate out and be inadvertently removed with the blood clot, giving the false impression of a negative cryoglobulin test. The blood should be allowed to clot at room temperature or in a warm bath (37°C) before it is sent for cryoglobulin testing. The presence of a cryoglobulin is considered abnormal and requires further evaluation by a specialist in immunology, hematology or oncology. Evaluation for a positive cryoglobulin test may include serum protein immunoelectrophoresis; immunofixation; T and B cell gene rearrangement with PCR amplification to detect occult T and/or B cell neoplasms; and hepatitis profiles. Hepatitis testing would be appropriate as some cryoglobulins are comprised of hepatitis antigen-antibody immune complexes.

- The diagnosis of **atypical cold urticaria** is more difficult because it cannot be confirmed by a direct cold stimulation test on the skin. The diagnosis can be confirmed only by replicating the same environmental cold conditions that induce symptoms. The patient should not take antihistamines for four days prior to this environmental cold challenge.

- The diagnosis of **familial cold auto-inflammatory syndrome** can be confirmed by a diagnostic genotype test for the cryopyrin gene using whole blood (EDTA). It can be tested at the laboratory of Hal Hoffman, M.D., (hahoffman@ucsd.edu). Symptomatic patients exhibit an elevation in the total white blood cell count and an abnormal differential with a marked shift to the left and elevated acute phase reactants.

- **Delayed cold urticaria** can be diagnosed by induction of a wheal several hours after performing a cold stimulation test.

#33. EXERCISE: H/S occurring during or after exercise is referred to as **exercise-induced anaphylaxis (EIA)**. H/S that occurs with exercise is associated with systemic symptoms of anaphylaxis characterized by nausea, vomiting, sweating, respiratory distress, low blood pressure, and loss of consciousness. When urticaria appears as part of this syndrome, it frequently affects the face, palms, and soles. The mechanism that causes exercise induction of urticaria is not fully understood. Ingestion of a normally tolerated food prior to or following exercise can trigger symptoms in some individuals. Any intensity of exercise, such as routine walking or vigorous running can induce episodes. Types of foods that have been associated with this disorder include shellfish, fish, wheat, celery, nuts, fruits, dairy products and alcohol.

Several theoretical mechanisms have been proposed to explain EIA.

- One mechanism suggests exercise and the associated increase in core body temperature may increase intestinal permeability, and thereby permit increased absorption of food allergens into the circulation. This mechanism suggests an individual may have a sub-threshold allergy to a food that is normally tolerated without exercise, but with exercise, there is rapid absorption and distribution of the food allergen, leading to an overt systemic reaction.

- Another theory proposes that exercise may cause an increase in endorphins. It is known that conventional opiates, such as morphine and codeine, can cause histamine release from mast cells. The theory suggests endorphins may also trigger histamine release, especially if mast cells are primed by a food allergen that has combined with its corresponding IgE antibodies.

- The occurrence of familial exercise-induced anaphylaxis **(#36B, chapter 5)** suggests genetic factors may also be involved.

- *In my experience, patients with a history of severe pollen-induced hay fever or asthma may develop H/S during exercise on days with high pollen counts. During exercise, larger quantities of pollen could be inhaled and rapidly absorbed through the respiratory tract into the circulation, causing systemic symptoms.*

Another exercise-induced urticaria condition is referred to as **cholinergic urticaria.** Most affected are male adolescents who break out with tiny, itchy hives during vigorous exercise. The urticaria may occur on most parts of the body except for the palms, soles and axillae. The mechanism for this condition is not understood, but clearly has some connection with an increase in core body temperature. There is speculation that affected individuals are sensitive to acetylcholine, which is released at neuro-muscular junctions during exercise.

RECOMMENDATIONS:
- An exercise test is advised for patients suspected of having **exercise-induced H/S**. Exercise testing should be performed on a treadmill under close medical supervision. **Equipment should be available to treat anaphylaxis.** The test should be discontinued at the earliest onset of H/S or anaphylaxis. Additional tests may include CBC, ESR, chemistry screen, allergy skin tests or IgE specific RAST tests for foods and inhalants, and beta tryptase. The latter is a mast cell marker which, if elevated, is diagnostic of anaphylaxis due to any cause. This test must be ordered within **two hours** of the onset of anaphylaxis in order to detect an elevated level.

- A skin test to an acetylcholine derivative, namely Mecholyl®, is advised if **cholinergic urticaria** is suspected. The diagnosis of cholinergic urticaria is confirmed if the skin test induces a wheal and erythema formation with a negative saline control. The Mecholyl challenge may be positive in only 30% of cases of cholinergic urticaria. Having patients run on a treadmill in warm clothing or in an occlusive training suit may provoke symptoms. On rare occasions, some patients with cholinergic urticaria can exhibit symptoms of anaphylaxis. Therefore, exercise challenges should be monitored under close medical supervision.

#34. BATHING OR SHOWERING IN WARM OR HOT WATER: Just as there are individuals who develop hives during cold exposure, there is a counterpart disorder in which individuals develop **heat-induced urticaria** from warm temperature exposure. The mechanism that causes this disorder is not understood. Typically, an individual will notice an outbreak of hives while bathing in warm or hot water, and in extreme circumstances, may experience anaphylactic symptoms with low blood pressure, loss of consciousness and shock. The onset of this disorder can be sudden and without warning.

RECOMMENDATIONS:

A heat test is advised for **heat-induced urticaria**. A glass filled with **tolerably** hot water is applied to the forearm for five minutes. After removal, allow the skin to return to normal body temperature and then determine whether a wheal has developed. The appearance of a wheal is a confirmation of heat-induced urticaria.

#35. CONTACT WITH WATER: Some individuals develop H/S when water of any temperature touches their skin. This condition is called **aquagenic urticaria**. No cause for this disorder is known.

RECOMMENDATIONS:

A provocation test is advised for **aquagenic urticaria**. The patient places an arm or hand under water for five minutes. After removal, inspect to determine whether wheals have developed. Testing is repeated at different locations using a range of water temperatures. The diagnosis of **aquagenic urticaria** is confirmed if H/S develops after exposure to all ranges of water temperature.

#36 THROUGH #42. FAMILY HISTORY OF H/S:

Several H/S disorders are inherited in an autosomal dominant pattern. The following hereditary conditions are associated with H/S:

#36. VIBRATORY ANGIOEDEMA is an autosomal dominant disorder in which individuals develop swelling after using vibrating tools or equipment, such as a jackhammer. No mechanism is known to explain how vibratory stimuli may cause these symptoms.

RECOMMENDATIONS:

The diagnosis can be confirmed by repeating the vibratory activity that induced the swelling.

#36A. FAMILIAL DERMOGRAPHISM is a dermographic disorder described in several families and is transmitted in an autosomal dominant manner.

RECOMMENDATIONS:

The diagnosis can be established by the procedures described in **(#30, chapter 5)**. HLA types A2, B16, A1 and B5 have been observed in one family with 25 affected members.

#36B. FAMILIAL EXERCISE-INDUCED ANAPHYLAXIS has been described in several generations involving at least two families. H/S can develop with anaphylaxis in this familial disorder. The pattern of inheritance is not understood.

RECOMMENDATIONS:

The diagnosis can be established by the procedures described in **(#33, chapter 5)**. One report describes a reduction in complement factors C_2 and C_5 during exercise.

#37. FAMILIAL COLD AUTO-INFLAMMATORY SYNDROME (PREVIOUSLY NAMED FAMILIAL COLD URTICARIA; #32, CHAPTER 5) is an autosomal dominant disorder characterized by the development of a rash, fever, and joint pains after cold exposure. Spontaneous mutations do occur, therefore a multi-generational family history is not necessary to consider the diagnosis. This genetic disorder is caused by mutations in a gene located on chromosome 1q44 that encodes proteins called cryopyrins.

RECOMMENDATIONS:

The diagnosis may require reproducing the conditions of cold exposure that have induced symptoms. Typically, a measles-like rash develops with fever and joint pains, all within a few hours after cold exposure. A CBC and ESR ordered at the peak of cold-induced symptoms will reveal a marked increase in the total white blood cell count, a shift to the left in the white blood cell differential, and an elevated ESR. The diagnosis of **familial cold auto-inflammatory syndrome** can be definitively confirmed by a diagnostic genotype test for the cryopyrin gene using whole blood (EDTA). It can be tested at the laboratory of Hal Hoffman, M.D. (hahoffman@ucsd.edu).

#38. DELAYED COLD URTICARIA (#32, CHAPTER 5) is a disorder with an autosomal dominant pattern of inheritance, characterized by the delayed onset of cold-induced urticaria. The mechanism that causes this disorder is unknown.

RECOMMENDATIONS:

A cold stimulation test (**#32, chapter 5**), is applied to the forearm for five minutes. The diagnosis is confirmed if a wheal develops several hours later.

#38A. FAMILIAL AQUAGENIC URTICARIA has been reported in three generations of one family in association with lactose intolerance.

RECOMMENDATIONS:

Direct contact with water of any temperature induces hives (**#35, chapter 5**). Lactose tolerance testing may also be indicated.

#39. HEREDITARY ANGIOEDEMA, (#26E, CHAPTER 5) is a disorder with an autosomal co-dominant pattern of inheritance. It is characterized by swelling triggered by mild traumatic procedures, such as dental treatments or tonsillectomy. Symptoms may also occur spontaneously without trauma induction. Swelling inside the mouth may be a life-threatening event and needs to be recognized and treated immediately. **Swelling associated with this hereditary condition never occurs with urticaria.** Therefore, this condition can be excluded if hives occur in combination with swelling. It is important to recognize that not all families with hereditary angioedema have a co-dominant autosomal pattern of inheritance as there are spontaneous mutations. The hereditary disorder is caused by a quantitative deficiency of C_1 esterase inhibitor (Type I), or a functional abnormality of the same protein (Type II). The same enzyme inhibitor is involved in the formation of blood clots and a deficiency in this inhibitor may increase bradykinin production, a mediator that may be responsible for swelling in these conditions. This condition is treatable **(#39, chapter 6)**.

RECOMMENDATIONS:

A decreased level of C_4 suggests the diagnosis and a decreased level of quantitative C_1 esterase inhibitor confirms it. Some hereditary angioedema patients (15%) have normal quantitative levels of C_1 esterase inhibitor with an abnormal functional assay of C_1 esterase inhibitor.

The acquired form has the same clinical appearance as the hereditary types. Decreased C_4 and C_{1q} levels are typically associated with the acquired type. Acquired angioedema with a decreased C_{1q} level can be associated with an abnormal functional assay of C_1 esterase inhibitor.

Further evaluation is required to search for a neoplasm if the C_{1q} level is low. These tests might include immunotyping of peripheral blood lymphocytes for the detection of malignant B cells; T and B cell gene rearrangement with PCR amplification to detect occult T and/or B cell neoplasms; serum protein immunoelectrophoresis and immunofixation to rule out dysproteinemia; and CT of the chest, abdomen, and pelvis to rule out a lymphoma or other neoplasm.

Acquired angioedema can also be caused by autoimmune disorders. If a neoplasm is not detected, an autoimmune evaluation is warranted and would include a test for autoantibody to C_1 esterase inhibitor and an ANA profile. Recent studies indicate some patients with autoantibodies to C_1 esterase inhibitor may eventually develop a malignant lymphoproliferative disease. Hence, continued surveillance for this possibility is advised.

Complement tests require the serum or EDTA plasma specimen be kept on dry ice during transportation.

#40. MUCKLE-WELLS SYNDROME is an autosomal dominant syndrome characterized by chronic nephrosis due to AA amyloidosis, occasional deafness, periodic fever and urticaria. It is caused by mutations on the same gene that is associated with Familial Cold Auto-inflammatory syndrome (**#32, chapter 5**). Interleukin-1 is thought to be involved as it contributes to increased synthesis of serum amyloid A.

RECOMMENDATIONS:

The diagnosis can be confirmed by a genotype test performed at the laboratory of Hal Hoffman, M.D. (E mail address: hahoffman@ucsd.edu.)

#41. HEREDITARY FEMALE HORMONE-DEPENDENT ANGIOEDEMA is a newly-described inherited disorder that affects only females in each generation. It affects pregnant women, or females who are receiving estrogen supplements or birth control medications. No cause for this disorder is known, other than the possibility that female hormones play a role.

RECOMMENDATIONS:

The diagnosis is based primarily on a history of swelling that affects only females in each generation. Patients do not have hives with this syndrome. Manifestations include laryngeal edema causing upper airway obstruction, and intestinal edema with abdominal pain. There does not appear to be involvement of the C_1 esterase inhibitor pathway.

#42 THROUGH #49. OCCUPATIONAL HISTORY; HOME HISTORY; RECREATIONAL HISTORY:

Occasionally **occupational exposure** is associated with the development of H/S.

The following are a few occupations that may be associated with H/S:

 # 42. HEALTHCARE WORK. H/S can be caused by blood borne infections, such as viral hepatitis or HIV, which are transmitted by sharp injuries or exposure to body fluids. These infections may cause H/S by immune complex formation and complement activation (**chapter 1; and "history of recent infection", #58, chapter 5**).

RECOMMENDATIONS:

The evaluation should include serological tests for hepatitis (A, B, and C) and HIV.

#43. LATEX EXPOSURE. Latex products can cause H/S and anaphylaxis. Exposure may occur in the healthcare profession, latex manufacturing, and with products that are not recognized as being latex. Allergic IgE antibodies to latex proteins cause H/S. Additionally, banana, kiwi, avocado and chestnut are cross-reacting foods that can increase sensitivity to latex.

RECOMMENDATIONS:

The diagnosis of latex sensitivity can be confirmed by an IgE RAST test to latex protein and by skin testing to latex protein prepared and tested by an experienced allergist. Since cross-reactive foods can increase sensitivity to latex, it is advisable to test for IgE antibodies to banana, kiwi, avocado and chestnut with skin tests or IgE RAST tests.

#44. ANIMAL CARE PROVIDERS. H/S is caused by allergic IgE antibodies to animal proteins.

RECOMMENDATIONS:

Animal sensitivity can be confirmed by immediate skin tests and/or IgE RAST tests.

OCCASIONALLY EXPOSURE TO ALLERGENS IN THE HOME ENVIRONMENT AND ACTIVITIES AT HOME MAY INDUCE H/S.

The following home-related exposures may be associated with H/S:

#45. ANIMAL EXPOSURE may cause H/S, such as cleaning a birdcage, or contact with a dog, cat, horse, cattle, or other animals. Allergic IgE antibodies to animal proteins cause H/S.

RECOMMENDATIONS:

Sensitivity to animals can be confirmed by immediate skin tests and/or IgE RAST tests.

#46. ARTS AND CRAFT MATERIALS can induce H/S, during or after direct contact with these materials. H/S can occur while handling chemical products, wools, glues, rubber, wood products, etc. The mechanism may be due to contact induction of allergic IgE antibodies.

RECOMMENDATIONS:

Testing for arts and crafts sensitivity is difficult, since most arts and craft chemicals and allergens are not available for conventional skin tests or RAST tests. Diluted topical products should be applied onto aluminum discs (Finn Chambers) when performing patch tests. The chambers can be purchased at Allerderm Company (Petaluma CA, www.allerderm.com). In general, it is advisable to dilute chemicals and products before patch testing to avoid severe irritant reactions. A good reference for proper patch test dilution is listed in the reference section (DeGroot AC, 1994). Common patch test chemicals and allergens can be ordered from Allerderm Inc. for use with T.R.U.E. test kits (Petaluma CA), and more unusual patch test chemicals can be ordered from Pharmascience Inc., (Montreal, Canada). A dermatologist or an allergist can also provide guidance. Patch tests to these materials should be read 30 minutes, 48 hours and 72 hours after application to detect immediate and delayed sensitivity reactions.

OCCASIONALLY RECREATIONAL ACTIVITIES MAY INDUCE H/S.

The following are recreational activities that may be associated with H/S:

#47. WATER ACTIVITIES OR COLD EXPOSURE can be associated with H/S.

RECOMMENDATIONS:
(**#32, #34, #35, chapter 5**).

#48. EXERCISE RELATED H/S.

RECOMMENDATIONS:
(**#33, chapter 5**)

#49. WEIGHT-LIFTING can induce delayed pressure urticaria.

RECOMMENDATIONS:
(**#30, chapter 5**)

#50. MEDICATION HISTORY: H/S is a common side effect associated with prescription or an over-the-counter medication. These symptoms are frequently listed as a side effect of most medications listed in the PDR (Physicians' Desk Reference). Consequently, it is essential that patients list all prescription and over- the-counter medications they are taking, medications stopped since onset of H/S, and all medications they have used during the month prior to onset of symptoms. The latter point is important to emphasize as drugs with long half-lives may cause H/S after they have been discontinued.

The medication list should include prescription medications, over-the-counter medications, including all herbal products, health supplements and vitamins. The list should also include oral medications, injections, products administered rectally or vaginally, topical applications on the skin, nasal and oral sprays, and ointments applied to the eyes or ears. I advise listing the ingredients of all products as part of this exercise and if possible taking all medications to the healthcare professional.

One example of an herbal product that causes H/S is bee pollen extract, which is sold as an oral remedy to prevent hay fever. Bee pollen product contains many varieties of pollen, including wind-borne pollens such as tree, grass and weeds. Persons sensitive to these pollens can develop life-threatening swelling inside the mouth and throat following ingestion of this product.

Hair shampoos and conditioners containing foreign animal protein and/or nettle extract can cause H/S around the eyes, face, and scalp. The nettle plant is legendary, as it can cause urticaria following direct contact with the plant. Its scientific name, *Urtica dioca*, reveals the urticaria potential of this plant.

Angiotensin converting enzyme inhibitors (ACE inhibitors, such as fosinopril (Monopril®), quinapril (Accupril®), captopril (Capoten®), and angiotensin II receptor antagonists (losartan; Cozaar®), prescribed for the treatment of hypertension, can cause swelling (angioedema). Angiotensin converting enzyme (ACE) is the same enzyme that catabolizes bradykinin. Consequently, ACE inhibitors may increase bradykinin concentrations that could cause swelling. ACE inhibitor-induced swelling may occur after beginning the drug, or after years of continuous use. There is a case report (Kleiner GI, 2002) in which swelling caused by ACE inhibitors unmasked acquired angioedema with a C_{1q} deficiency.

All anti-inflammatory drugs such as aspirin, ibuprofen, naprosyn and related medications can cause or flare up H/S. It is not unusual for an individual to take aspirin unsuspectingly in over-the-counter medications, such as in Alka-Seltzer®, because it is listed by its chemical name, acetylsalicylic acid. This is another example of why all medications need to be listed.

The documentation of antimicrobial sensitivity is very difficult because there are no reliable blood tests. Skin testing is not a standardized procedure except for some penicillin tests. Some old rules for predicting tolerance to antibiotics are being challenged. In the past, if a patient developed an allergy to penicillin, one could generally assume that the same patient would tolerate a different class of antibiotic.

Patients have been described (Sullivan, 1991) who have a propensity to antibiotic drug allergy that is not confined to a single class of drug. It is unclear whether this proclivity for multiple-drug sensitivity is a genetically-determined phenomenon or related to some acquired immune dysfunction.

Intravenous drugs such as radiocontrast media are occasionally associated with H/S.

RECOMMENDATIONS:

CBC, ESR, and chemistry screen may suggest a drug is causing hypersensitivity effects which are not clinically recognized.

- **Drug hypersensitivity** may cause an elevated eosinophil count. A hypersensitivity reaction to a drug may involve the liver and cause elevations of liver enzymes.

- Unfortunately, there are no reliable **blood tests** that can diagnose sensitivity to a particular medication. RAST IgE tests may be obtained for penicillin and amoxicillin, but these tests may give false negative results. Skin testing may be considered as an alternative in those circumstances (see below).

- A **total complement CH$_{50}$** might be included in the evaluation. Decreased total complement might suggest an immune complex-mediated hypersensitivity reaction (i.e. serum sickness) to a drug. Further tests might include immune complex assays (Raji equivalent C$_{3D}$ assay, solid C$_{1q}$ assay). Complement tests require the serum or EDTA plasma specimen be kept on dry ice during transportation.

- On occasion, allergists can perform **skin tests with some medications**, although testing is not routinely standardized. Testing for **penicillin** allergy requires skin testing to two types of penicillin antigens, the major determinants, which represent the higher concentration of penicillin metabolites, and the minor determinants, which represent the smaller concentration of penicillin metabolites. The major determinants of penicillin can be tested with a commercial product called benzylpenicilloyl polylysine (Pre-pen®, manufactured by Hollister-Stier). A positive

Pre-pen® skin test correlates with the potential for induction of H/S by penicillin. The minor determinants are antigens that have the potential to produce anaphylaxis. Unfortunately, no commercial product is available to test for the minor antigens. Allergists can prepare minor determinant antigen mixtures with penicillin G that has been incubated at room temperature for two to three days. The obvious concern is that these preparations are not standardized for minor determinant concentrations.

- **Skin testing for other drugs** has not been standardized. Some allergists make dilutions of aqueous-based drugs and perform skin puncture tests, followed by intradermal testing. Some drug testing is unreliable because certain types of drugs, such as opiates, can cause H/S in everyone tested due to the direct degranulation of mast cells.

  Careful skin testing can be used with patients presumed to be allergic to vaccines. This approach still requires cautious subcutaneous challenges using diluted vaccine preparations. (Barbaud, 1998; Georgitis JW, 2001).

- **Skin care products** suspected of causing H/S can be **patch tested** by applying diluted topical products onto aluminum discs called Finn Chambers. These can be purchased at Allerderm Company (Petaluma CA, www.allerderm.com). It is advisable to dilute chemicals and products before patch testing to avoid severe irritant reactions. Allerderm can provide information on the appropriate dilutions for testing common topical products. A good reference for proper patch test dilution is listed in the reference section (DeGroot AC, 1994). Common patch test chemicals and allergens can be ordered from Allerderm Inc. for use with T.R.U.E. test kits (Petaluma CA). More unusual patch test chemicals can be ordered from Pharmascience Inc. (Montreal, Canada). A dermatologist or allergist can also provide guidance. Patch tests to these materials should be read 30 minutes, 48 hours, and 72 hours after application to detect immediate and delayed sensitivity reactions .

There is one screening test that can be used to test cosmetics, lotions, shampoos and other healthcare products normally used on skin. Apply a single product behind one knee and in the flexion area of one elbow. A healthcare professional should read the areas at 30 minutes, 48 hours, and 72 hours after application. A skin response is considered positive if redness, itching, or wheals develop, providing the untested similar skin areas are unaffected. Use of the tested product should be discontinued if any of these reactions occur.

- As previously mentioned, **ACE inhibitors** and **angiotensin II receptor antagonists** may cause angioedema. Since ACE inhibitors can also unmask acquired angioedema due to C_1 esterase inhibitor defects, it may be advisable to order a C_{1q}. If the latter is decreased, evaluate the patient for a malignant lymphoproliferative disease (**#76, chapter 5**) or an autoimmune disorder involving the presence of autoantibodies to C_1 esterase inhibitor (**#91A, chapter 5**).

#51. INSECT HISTORY: Insect bites and stings can cause H/S. The most common insect bites or stings that induce H/S are bees, fire ants, ticks, mosquitoes and deer flies. H/S reactions resulting from insect stings and bites are usually classified as acute, because they persist for six weeks or less.

The most common stinging insects of the *Hymenoptera* class which cause H/S and systemic anaphylactic reactions are the honey bee, yellow jacket, wasp and hornet. The fire ant is related to bee species and it may cause similar clinical reactions. Currently, test materials for bees and fire ant are available, but there are no reliable test materials for ticks, mosquitoes, deer flies and other insects.

RECOMMENDATIONS:

Testing is indicated if H/S is generalized and not localized to the site of the bee sting, or if signs of a systemic reaction occur, such as dizziness, loss of consciousness, difficult swallowing or breathing, wheezing, generalized flushing, or shock.

- Workup for H/S and systemic reactions may include RAST tests for venom specific IgE allergic antibody to the suspect bee or fire ant. It is important to request venom-specific IgE antibody measurements to confirm sensitivity to the suspect venom. These tests should not be confused with venom-specific IgG antibody tests that reflect levels of antibody protection following bee venom immunotherapy. It is imperative to order all bee venom-specific IgE RAST tests, if the type of bee sting cannot be identified. Patients with elevated venom-specific IgE antibodies should be referred to an allergist for further evaluation and treatment. The allergist will most likely recommend skin tests to the suspect insect venoms in order to document the level of sensitivity and to determine the beginning dose of venom immunotherapy.

- An elevated serum beta tryptase would provide substantive evidence that a bee sting has caused a systemic reaction. This test must be ordered within **two hours** of the bee sting in order to detect an elevated level. This would be an indication for venom immunotherapy.

#52. FOOD HISTORY: Immediate induction of H/S after the ingestion of a food is generally easy to recognize. Foods that frequently cause these reactions are dairy products; egg; peanut and other tree nuts, such as walnut and cashew; fish; shellfish; soy and wheat. Direct skin contact with a food or food-contaminated utensil can cause immediate H/S. Kissing someone who has recently ingested a food allergen may cause immediate H/S involving lips, mouth and other contacted areas.

The more difficult problem is identifying a relationship between chronic H/S and foods. Reviewing the background issues on this subject in **chapter 1** will help to understand why it is difficult to prove food causation of chronic H/S.

RECOMMENDATIONS:

- Skin tests and IgE RAST tests to foods and/or food dyes may be appropriate if the history is suggestive of a relationship between ingesting a food/food dye and the development of H/S. An interesting case report (Keitel D, 2002) describes a patient who developed chronic hives from sensitivity to dyes in colored candies. In this report, skin tests to dyes induced positive wheal and flare responses and generalized hives that required treatment with epinephrine. Skin test materials for food dyes can be obtained from Hollister-Stier Laboratories (Spokane, WA).

- Ordering a beta tryptase blood level is advised if H/S is associated with symptoms suggestive of anaphylaxis, such as shock reactions, flushing, difficulty breathing, and loss of consciousness. An elevated beta tryptase level suggests H/S was part of a systemic allergic reaction. This test must be ordered within **two hours** following the onset of symptoms in order to detect an elevated level. Unfortunately, some cases of food-induced anaphylaxis may be associated with a normal beta tryptase level.

- More often the history is not suggestive of a relationship between foods and H/S. In this circumstance testing using multiple skin tests or IgE RAST tests is not advised, since false positive and false negative results are produced which may not correlate with the history. Moreover, the probability of finding a causative food is highly unlikely.

- There are several approaches that may be more effective:

  - The first is to ask the patient to keep a detailed diary for one to three weeks that includes columns for time of day and night, foods ingested, activities, and medications. Rating of hives should be recorded when there is an increase in severity and graded from 0 to 4: 0= no hives; 1= 1 to 5 hives; 2= 6 to 10 hives; 3= 11 to 20 hives; 4= more than 20 hives. Swelling severity can also be rated using a similar scale: 0= no swelling; 1= 1 swelling; 2= 2 swellings; 3= 3 swellings; and 4= 4 or more swellings. This is just an example of a severity rating scale, which can be personalized by the patient or the healthcare professional (**Appendix 2**). The ingredients of foods ingested should also be detailed and listed. The healthcare professional can review the diary to determine whether there is a causative relationship between foods and H/S.

  - A second approach is an elimination diet in which the affected person starts with basic foods such as organic rice, lamb and water for seven to ten days.

If the H/S ceases, one food is added every three days. If H/S recurs, the suspect food is eliminated and then added again two or three weeks later. If the same response occurs, the food in question is permanently eliminated. If the H/S has not ceased after a seven to ten day trial on this diet, it is highly unlikely that H/S is caused by a food or food additive.

As of October 2002, the USDA requires food products be labeled as 100% ORGANIC if they contain only organic ingredients without additives, hormones, dyes, etc. Although expensive, ingesting only organic foods may be a good test of whether additives play a role in H/S induction.

- A third approach is to stop eating all foods and place the patient on a diet of an elementary balanced food product comprised of basic amino acids, simple carbohydrates and digested fats (Pregestimil®; Tolerex®; Vivonex®) for seven to ten days. One food can be added every three days, as previously described. It is highly unlikely that H/S is caused by a food or food additive if the H/S has not ceased after this trial.

- A fourth approach is to perform challenge tests with suspect foods, which should be done carefully and monitored by a healthcare professional. Ideally to make objective observations, the challenge should be blinded so neither the patient nor the healthcare professional know whether the patient is receiving the challenge food or placebo. One important issue related to this approach is being sure to challenge with the same food preparation (cooked, uncooked, etc.) that was associated with the clinical response.

- There are some cautions on food tests that claim to accurately detect food allergy. Consumers need to be aware most commercial food tests are notoriously inaccurate and scientifically unproven. **The American Academy of Allergy, Asthma, and Immunology has a position paper (Ann Allergy Asthma Immunol 1995 Dec;75 (6Pt2): 543-625) on all but kinesiology testing and has declared them to be INVALID predictors of food allergy:**

  - Cytotoxic blood test: This test is performed by adding a food allergen to a blood specimen and inspecting for white blood cell alteration, which is claimed to be indicative of food allergy.

- Provocative and neutralization testing using oral and injection techniques. These methods involve the injection of a food allergen subcutaneously into the skin or the application of food drops under the tongue to elicit symptoms corresponding to patients' complaints. This is followed by the injection or oral drop administration of the same food allergen at a weaker strength to relieve symptoms.

- Pulse tests: These tests are based on the unfounded claim that food allergy can be detected by monitoring pulse rate increases after ingesting a food.

- Kinesiology tests: These tests are based on the unfounded claim that food allergy can be detected by changes in muscle strength. The NAET method involves placing a food in the patient's hand and pulling down on their flexed arm to test for muscle weakness. The patient is claimed to be allergic to that food if arm weakness is detected. There is no position paper on this technique to date. One can read critically about this technique by accessing the following medical site: (http://www.chirobase.org/06DD/naet.html)

- RAST IgG antibodies: These tests are based on the unfounded claim that elevated IgG_1 and IgG_4 antibodies are indicative of food allergy. Most individuals exhibit positive food IgG RAST tests, and the results do not correlate with clinical evidence of food allergy or other disease states. These tests should not be confused with RAST tests that detect IgE allergic antibodies to foods.

All of the aforementioned tests are unproven methods and should not be relied on to predict food allergy. IgE RAST tests are legitimate blood tests considered equivalent to skin tests for the detection of IgE antibodies to a food. However, IgE RAST and skin tests can produce false negative and false positive results and consequently should be used only as a guideline in the management of food allergy problems. The Food Allergy and Anaphylaxis Network is a good resource to learn more about foods and H/S. The web site address is :http://www.foodallergy.org

#53. TRAVEL HISTORY: People who travel can be exposed to parasitic infections, viral hepatitis and other infectious illnesses. These infections are commonly acquired by ingesting contaminated foods and liquids. Some parasitic and viral infections are transmitted through insect bites. Diarrhea, nausea, vomiting, fever, severe headaches, joint pains, and fatigue may precede or accompany H/S, which is caused by an infection acquired during foreign travel.

H/S with viral hepatitis may be caused by immune complex formation and complement activation (**chapter 1**). Similar mechanisms may be operative for other acquired infectious illnesses.

The parasite, *Giardia lamblia*, is the most common parasite acquired in the U.S and has been reported to cause H/S. It is transmitted by the ingestion of water contaminated with deer or animal fecal matter containing this parasite. *Giardia* can be transmitted in contaminated water from a well, river, pond, lake or other unpurified water sources.

No mechanism is known to explain the occurrence of H/S and parasitic infestations, although it is tempting to consider that H/S is caused by an abnormal immune response to parasites, such as activation of complement (**chapter 1 and "history of recent infection" #58, chapter 5**) or an immediate IgE antibody-mediated sensitivity to a parasitic allergen (**chapter 1**).

RECOMMENDATIONS:

- CBC, total eosinophil count, ESR, chemistry screen, hepatitis profiles for types A, B and C, total complement CH_{50}, IgE and several stool examinations for ova and parasites. Elevated eosinophil counts and IgE levels may be suggestive of a parasitic infection. Serological tests, such as serum antibodies to *Strongyloides* and *Trichinella*, may be ordered in the event parasitic disease is an important consideration. A decreased total complement level might suggest an immune complex-mediated disease, which can be documented via immune complex assays (Raji equivalent C_{3D} assay, solid C_{1q} assay).

Complement tests require the serum or EDTA plasma specimen be kept on dry ice during transportation.

- Suspicion of a *Giardia* infection may require an upper intestinal aspirate of the duodenum to search for this parasite.

#54 THROUGH #57: HORMONE HISTORY: H/S can be induced or associated with an assortment of hormonal disorders.

GENERAL RECOMMENDATIONS FOR HORMONE HISTORY:
CBC and chemistry screen.

54, #55. DISORDERS OF THE THYROID GLAND: AUTOIMMUNE INFLAMMATION OF THE THYROID, I.E. THYROIDITIS, can initially cause **hyperthyroidism** (# 55), with symptoms of increased metabolism manifested by rapid pulse, prominent eyes, weight loss, irregular menstrual cycles, sweating, heat intolerance, tremors, enlarged neck, and possibly lumps in the neck. As thyroiditis progresses, the thyroid gland may exhaust itself leading to **hypothyroidism** (#54) with symptoms of low metabolism, such as fatigue, weight gain, hair loss, puffiness around the eyes, low pulse rate, irregular menstrual cycles, cold intolerance, dry skin, enlarged neck, and possibly lumps in the neck. For unknown reasons, autoimmune thyroiditis (Hashimoto's disease) can be associated with chronic H/S. Autoantibodies to thyroid can be detected in this disorder. Treatment of thyroiditis with replacement thyroid hormone may control H/S, even when thyroid levels are normal (**#54 in Chapter 6, Part B III**). Primary hyperthyroidism without thyroiditis (Grave's disease) may also cause H/S.

RECOMMENDATIONS:

A thyroid screen (free T_4, TSH, and perioxidase/thyroglobulin anti-thyroid antibodies) is indicated for low and high thyroid conditions caused by autoimmune thyroiditis and Grave's disease.

#56. HYPERPARATHYROIDISM can be associated with H/S (# 24, chapter 5). Manifestations of an overactive parathyroid gland may be a lump in the neck, frequent bone fractures and kidney stones. An overactive parathyroid gland can cause H/S, possibly because it can elevate calcium levels, which may lead to histamine and mediator release from mast cells.

RECOMMENDATIONS:

Total calcium, ionized calcium, parathyroid hormone and parathyroid hormone-related protein (PTHrP) would be appropriate.

#57. H/S COINCIDING WITH MENSTRUAL CYCLES. Occasionally, a female patient may notice that H/S recurs monthly with her menstrual cycle. The cause of this condition is not understood, although there is speculation it is caused by sensitivity to progesterone. Symptoms of anaphylaxis may be associated with this disorder (**#92, chapter 5**).

RECOMMENDATIONS:

Skin tests with aqueous progesterone or an analog (medroxyprogesterone) may detect allergic IgE antibodies to these hormones. Aqueous progesterone in saline should be tested intradermally at a concentration of 0.1 mg/ml and if necessary, with an intradermal test of 1 mg/ml. Skin testing with medroxyprogesterone should be performed cautiously as anaphylaxis has been reported when testing with this compound.

#57A. A SECOND TYPE OF H/S COINCIDING WITH THE MENSTRUAL CYCLE is characterized by urticaria occurring at the end of the menstrual cycle and is associated with elevated eosinophil counts and decreased levels of progesterone.

RECOMMENDATIONS:

Total eosinophil counts and serum progesterone levels should be obtained while the patient is symptomatic. Elevated eosinophil counts occurring with decreased progesterone levels may suggest the disorder of cyclic urticaria with hypereosinophilia.

#57B. HEREDITARY ESTROGEN-DEPENDENT ANGIOEDEMA is a newly described inherited disorder that affects only pregnant women, or females who are receiving either estrogen supplements or birth control medications (**#41, chapter 5**). No cause for this disorder is known, other than the possibility estrogens play a causative role. Hives do not occur with this syndrome. Other manifestations of swelling include laryngeal edema with upper airway obstruction, and intestinal edema that causes abdominal pain. There does not appear to be involvement of the C_1 esterase inhibitor pathway.

RECOMMENDATIONS:

The history can confirm the diagnosis of **hereditary estrogen-dependent angioedema**, in which affected women develop swelling while on estrogen supplements, birth control pills, or during pregnancy. A C_4 would be useful to screen for hereditary angioedema caused by quantitative C_1 esterase inhibitor deficiency or functional abnormalities of the C_1 esterase inhibitor.

#57C. PRURITIC URTICARIAL PAPULES AND PLAQUES OF PREGNANCY (PUPPP) is a skin disorder associated with pregnancy characterized by papular hives, erythema and plaques. It may affect any part of the body, but the hives typically spare the face, palms and soles. It is a self-limiting disorder that usually disappears after pregnancy.

RECOMMENDATIONS:

There is no diagnostic test and the diagnosis is primarily based on clinical appearance.

#58. HISTORY OF RECENT INFECTION: The acute form of H/S can be caused by infectious illnesses, such as viral respiratory infections in children, parasitic infections, HIV, viral hepatitis, infectious mononucleosis and other infectious diseases.

There is scant scientific evidence to support the concept that chronic H/S can be caused by infectious illnesses, other than isolated case reports describing the association of chronic H/S with specific infections, such as sinus infections, streptococcal infections, and viral hepatitis.

Occasionally a case report can be supportive of the notion that infections may cause chronic H/S. One such report (Ostrov MR, 1995) described a young woman who experienced chronic H/S for several years. She had hemorrhoid surgery several months prior to the onset of H/S. The H/S was a continuous management problem over a three-year period requiring trials with combinations of antihistamines and steroids. A draining, infected fistula was subsequently discovered near the location of the original surgical procedure. A second surgical procedure was required to repair and treat the draining wound. The chronic H/S completely resolved following the second procedure. There was one laboratory clue that may have suggested the existence of the unrecognized chronic bacterial infection in this patient, namely a decreased total complement CH_{50} level. Reduction in complement levels can reflect immune complex formation, which can cause production of biologically active products, namely, anaphylatoxins that release histamine and other chemical mediators from mast cells. The mediators and their biologic effects, in turn, may cause H/S. Unfortunately, there is no large series of similar cases, so the medical profession remains skeptical about the possibility that chronic infection causes chronic H/S.

Another mechanism has been proposed (Boyce JA, 2003) to explain microbe activation of mast cells. Studies reveal that mast cells have receptors (called toll receptors) which recognize patterns of microbial antigens. These receptors are recognized by microbes which then activate mast cells without involvement of pre-existing immune mechanisms, such as antibody production. The end effect is microbial generation of mediators that induce or exacerbate inflammatory responses. A wide spectrum of microbes may cause mast cell activation by this mechanism, including common respiratory viruses. This observation explains outbreaks of presumed viral-induced urticaria in pediatric populations, as well as the induction of urticaria and angioedema by various infectious agents.

More recently, a medical report (Altshul et al, 2002) described the association of common variable immunodeficiency (CVID) and H/S in 6 patients. Several patients with H/S had a history of recurring respiratory infections. This report raises the interesting question of whether immunoglobulin levels should be measured in patients with chronic idiopathic H/S and a history of repeated infections.

I remain undecided about the relationship between infections and chronic H/S and believe an open mind is essential in working up these patients with H/S. Consequently, I have included questions relevant to infectious illnesses in the history questionnaire. It is not within the scope of this section to list every known symptom or sign of infectious illnesses. I will be referring to the more common indicators that might signify the coexistence of an infectious disease with H/S.

GENERAL RECOMMENDATIONS:

CBC, ESR, mono test, chemistry screen, quantitative immunoglobulin, specific diagnostics (X-rays, cultures) and total complement CH_{50}. If the total complement CH_{50} level is decreased, other complement-related tests might be appropriate, such as anaphylatoxin detection by measuring complement-activated products (C_{5a}, C_{5b}, C_{4a}). Immune complex assays (Raji equivalent C_{3D} assay, and solid C_{1q} assay) may also be considered, if the CH_{50} level is decreased.

Complement tests require the serum or EDTA plasma specimen be kept on dry ice during transportation.

The following includes examples of infectious illnesses and other conditions sometimes associated with H/S:

#58A. FEVER in combination with chronic H/S essentially rules out classic IgE-mediated allergy as a cause of H/S, since allergic mechanisms are typically not associated with fever. The presence of fever may suggest the co-existence of an infectious disease process. Acute or chronic viral illnesses can be associated with the onset of H/S. One particularly interesting association is acute infectious mononucleosis, which may induce acquired cold urticaria (**# 32, chapter 5**). Fever should be considered a non-specific symptom, as it may also be associated with non-infectious inflammatory disease processes, such as autoimmune diseases and serum sickness (**#9, chapter 5, for discussion of other causes of fever with hives**). Fever with weight gain, urticaria, angioedema, eosinophilia, elevated IgM and leukocytosis may suggest the syndrome of episodic angioedema with eosinophilia (**#10, chapter 5**). Nevertheless, persistent fever with H/S should be noted and worked up for the detection of an infectious disease.

RECOMMENDATIONS:

A **fever** evaluation can be minimal or very extensive. The healthcare professional should determine which tests are required for this evaluation.

#58B. RECURRING RESPIRATORY TRACT INFECTIONS AND UNUSUAL INFECTIONS in combination with H/S may signify an underlying immunodeficiency disorder, such as common variable immunodeficiency (CVID). This disorder is characterized by repeated bacterial infections involving the respiratory tract (lungs, sinuses, middle ear) and can be responsible for end stage lung disease (COPD, bronchiectasis). Infections of other systems may be involved, particularly the gastrointestinal tract and skin (furunculosis). Typically serum IgG, IgA and IgM levels are decreased by 2 standard deviations below the mean for age. Occasionally, T cell abnormalities are noted. There is an increased incidence of systemic autoimmune disease associated with CVID.

RECOMMENDATIONS:

A screening approach for **CVID** is advised: CBC, chemistry screen, quantitative immunoglobulin and ANA panel. Further tests may be required to assess humoral and/or cell-mediated immunity. An allergist-clinical immunologist may be of assistance.

#59. VIRAL HEPATITIS. Patients with H/S should be evaluated for **viral hepatitis** if they develop **jaundice**, are exposed to persons with hepatitis, or are considered to be at high risk for acquiring hepatitis. Viral hepatitis may cause H/S due to immune complex formation and complement activation (**chapter 1**).

RECOMMENDATIONS:

An evaluation for **jaundice** or the possibility of **hepatitis** infection may include liver function tests and viral hepatitis profiles for types A, B, and C.

#60, #61. SORE THROAT is another non-specific symptom that may occur in combination with H/S. This symptom may be associated with **infectious mononucleosis,** and **throat or sinus infections** caused by viral and bacterial agents. The potential relationship of infection with H/S has been previously discussed (**chapter 1, and "history of recent infection" #58, chapter 5**). Additionally, sore throat could be a manifestation of **angioedema** that involves the pharynx and uvula.

RECOMMENDATIONS:

The workup of **sore throat** in combination with H/S may include a streptococcal throat culture, streptozyme titer, and a test for infectious mononucleosis. Chronic sore throat can be a manifestation of post-nasal drainage from a sinus infection and consequently, a sinus infection workup may be indicated (sinus X-ray or limited CT scan of the sinuses). Angioedema screening might include C_4 and C_{1q} measurements.

 # 62. COLD SORES may be a manifestation of chronic Herpes Simplex virus infection that can cause erythema multiforme (**Appendix 1**). This syndrome may be difficult to differentiate from urticaria.

RECOMMENDATIONS:

Recurring **cold sores** would suggest possible Herpes Simplex virus infection that may require viral cultures or specific antibody blood titers obtained at baseline and at three to four weeks after the onset of symptoms.

#63. DRAINING BACTERIAL WOUNDS. The coexistence of a **draining bacterial wound** with H/S should be evaluated. The case report in "**history of recent infection**" **#58, chapter 5**, underscores the possible relationship between chronic bacterial infections and H/S.

RECOMMENDATIONS:

A **draining wound** should be evaluated by the healthcare professional and cultured for infectious organisms. Other diagnostics may be required, as noted in **#58, chapter 5**.

#64. INFECTION OF THE SINUSES has been anecdotally described with H/S. Sinus infections can present with any of the following symptoms: discolored nasal drainage, sore throat, facial tenderness, headaches, foul breath, loss of smell or taste, and fever. Chronic sinus infections may coexist without any clinical symptoms or signs. The case report in "**history of recent infection**" **#58, chapter 5**, underscores the possible relationship between chronic bacterial infections and H/S. The possibility of an immune deficiency must also be considered, such as common variable immunodeficiency (CVID), which exhibits decreased levels of IgG, IgM and IgA.

RECOMMENDATIONS:

A history of discolored nasal drainage may suggest the need for a **sinus infection** workup (sinus X-ray or limited CT scan of the sinuses) and quantitative immuno-globulins.

#65. GINGIVITIS OR DENTAL ABSCESS: Recent history of gingivitis or dental abscesses has been reported to cause H/S. The case report in "**history of recent infection**" **#58, chapter 5,** underscores the possible relationship between chronic bacterial infections and H/S.

RECOMMENDATIONS:

A dental evaluation would be appropriate.

#66. ASSOCIATION OF A BACTERIAL INFECTION (*Helicobacter pylori*) IN THE STOMACH OR UPPER GASTROINTESTINAL TRACT AND H/S. This association has not been scientifically proven as available data are contradictory. Nevertheless, it may be advisable to evaluate for H. *pylori* infection in H/S patients with coexisting stomach or duodenal ulcers, or symptoms of an ulcer such as abdominal pain, heartburn, nausea, vomiting, tarry stools, unexplained cough or reflux of acid secretions. No mechanism is known to explain the unproven association of H. *pylori* with H/S.

RECOMMENDATIONS:

Stomach symptoms (abdominal pain, acid reflux, heartburn, and cough) accompanying H/S may suggest the need for an H. *pylori* workup. Tests may include an IgG antibody blood test for H. *pylori*, C urea breath test, upper GI series and possibly, endoscopy.

#67. CHOLECYSTITIS: There is sparse medical literature to support the claim that H/S can be caused by **cholecystitis**. Symptoms of gall bladder infection may include abdominal pain, especially in the upper right quadrant of the abdomen, nausea after eating fatty foods, and fever. Jaundice can occur if a loose gallstone blocks a bile duct in the liver. The case report in "**history of recent infection**" **#58, chapter 5,** under-scores the possible relationship between chronic bacterial infections and H/S.

RECOMMENDATIONS:

A history of gall bladder symptoms suggesting **cholecystitis** may necessitate a cholecystogram and/or ultrasound study to rule out gallstones.

#68. FUNGAL INFECTIONS: ("ATHLETE'S FOOT"). A few reports claim athlete's foot or other fungal infections of the skin may cause H/S. There is no known mechanism to explain the unproven association of athlete's foot and H/S.

RECOMMENDATIONS:

Inflammation in the webs of toes may suggest a chronic infection with **fungi**. Fungal infections can affect other parts of the body, such as hands, under arms and groin. Workup may include scraping inflamed skin for KOH examination with microscopy and culture for fungal organisms.

#69. SKIN INFECTIONS AND ABSCESSES have been reported to cause H/S. The case report in "**history of recent infection**" **#58, chapter 5,** underscores the possible relationship between chronic bacterial infections and H/S. The possibility of an immune deficiency must also be considered, such as common variable immunode-ficiency (CVID), with decreased levels of IgG, IgM and IgA.

RECOMMENDATIONS:

Cultures for bacteria and quantitative immunoglobulins.

#70. YEAST INFECTIONS: It is claimed **yeast infections** (mouth, gastrointestinal tract, vagina, etc.) produce toxins that can cause H/S. This concept, which remains scientifically unproven, is referred to as the yeast or *Candida* theory and has been promoted in several books.

RECOMMENDATIONS:

Yeast infections can be confirmed with fungal cultures.

#71. INFECTIONS OF THE RESPIRATORY TRACT have been associated with H/S. The case report in "**history of recent infection**" **#58, chapter 5**, underscores the possible relationship between chronic bacterial infections and H/S. The possibility of an immune deficiency must also be considered, such as common variable immunodeficiency (CVID), with decreased levels of IgG, IgM and IgA.

RECOMMENDATIONS:

The evaluation of recurring or persistent **bronchial infections** may include a chest X-ray, sputum cultures for infectious organisms, quantitative immunoglobulins and basic pulmonary function tests.

#72. INFECTIONS OF THE URINARY TRACT have been associated with H/S. The case report in "**history of recent infection**" **#58, chapter 5,** underscores the possible relationship between chronic bacterial infections and H/S.

RECOMMENDATIONS:

Urine analysis and urine cultures.

#73. SEXUALLY TRANSMITTED INFECTIONS can be associated with chronic H/S. Several case studies have reported the development of H/S following infections with HIV, syphilis, gonococcus, and trichomonas.

RECOMMENDATIONS:

A workup for **sexually transmitted diseases** might include blood tests for syphilis, HIV, hepatitis profile, and cultures of genital secretions.

#74, #75. HISTORY OF NEEDLE STICKS OR TRANSFUSIONS. There is convincing medical evidence that **viral hepatitis** (A, B, C) and other blood-borne infections may cause H/S. Patients who develop H/S following transfusions or needle-sticks should be evaluated for this possibility.

RECOMMENDATIONS:

Appropriate tests include liver function tests, viral hepatitis profiles for types A, B, and C, and HIV tests.

#76. HISTORY OF TUMORS, CANCERS: The association of cancer with H/S is almost exclusively based on case reports (see reference section **"cancer"**). There is also literature challenging the validity of this association. All types of cancers have been reported with H/S. They include lymphomas, leukemias, gammopathies, and solid tumors affecting the brain, thyroid gland, lung, colon, testicles, ovaries and skin. Examples of H/S associated with cancers include chronic lymphoid leukemia with acquired cold urticaria, and acquired angioedema in association with underlying lymphoma, chronic lymphocytic leukemia and/or solid tumors. The suggestion that cancer may cause H/S is bolstered by case reports that describe resolution of H/S after surgical removal of neoplasms and/or following chemotherapy. There are no accepted mechanisms that explain the occurrence of H/S with cancers. Symptoms of co-existing cancer can include fatigue, low grade fever, weight loss, appetite change, unexplained swellings or lumps, prolonged or recurring bleeding at any location, changes in the color of skin lesions, chronic ulcers of the skin, or a new symptom involving any body system, such as a cough, change in bowel habits, or blood in the urine. It is beyond the scope of this book to include every symptom, sign or cancer that has been reported with H/S.

GENERAL RECOMMENDATIONS:

CBC, ESR, chemistry screen, serum protein immunoelectrophoresis and immunofixation, and appropriate X-rays. The healthcare professional should determine the need for cancer screening such as, breast and pelvic examination, mammogram, Pap smear and PSA test.

- Evaluation for **occult lymphoma or solid neoplasm** may be indicated for individuals who develop angioedema for no apparent reason. Appropriate tests for **acquired angioedema** may include CT scans of the chest, abdomen and pelvis, C_4, and C_{1q}. The latter two measurements are typically decreased in acquired angioedema. Immunophenotyping of peripheral blood lymphocytes; T and B cell gene rearrangement with PCR amplification to detect occult T and/or B cell neoplasms; and serum immunofixation may also be indicated. Angioedema patients with consistently decreased C_{1q} levels should be followed long term, as lymphomas may be detected many years after the onset of angioedema.

- Hypercalcemia and hypophosphatemia may occur with occult cancers of the lung and kidney in which bone metastases are absent or not clinically detectable. A malignancy-related parathyroid hormone-related protein (PTHrp) may induce hypercalcemia that could cause urticaria. A workup for occult malignancy might also include calcium, phosphorus, parathyroid hormone and PTHrp.

#77 through #83. HISTORY OF ENVIRONMENTAL EXPOSURE THROUGH DIRECT SKIN CONTACT: There are many examples of environmental exposure that can cause contact H/S. The mechanisms may be IgE-mediated and in some cases, the contact substance can cause hives through direct release of histamine and other mediators. Examples of the latter would be nettle plants; jellyfish; antibiotics, such as polymyxin and bacitracin; and some insect venoms.

#77. CONTACT WITH PLANTS such as nettle plants, celery plants, noxious weeds, and cedar bushes may cause H/S. There is no general mechanism to explain these occurrences, although plant toxin exposure may cause non-immune release of mediators from mast cells (**chapter 1**). IgE antibody-mediated mechanisms may also be involved.

RECOMMENDATIONS:
Exposure to any of these **plant** substances may require tests to detect IgE sensitivity to specific allergens. These tests would include conventional allergy skin tests, IgE RAST tests and/or patch tests read 30 minutes after the application of the test substances.

- Diluted topical plant extracts should be applied onto aluminum discs (Finn Chambers) when performing patch tests. The chambers can be purchased at Allerderm Company (Petaluma CA, www.allerderm.com). In general, it is advisable to dilute plant extracts before patch testing to avoid severe irritant reactions. A good reference for proper patch test dilution is listed in the reference section (DeGroot AC, 1994). Some plant extracts and allergens for patch testing can be ordered from Pharmascience Inc. (Montreal, Canada). A dermatologist or allergist can also provide guidance.

#78. CONTACT WITH ANIMALS: Individuals who are sensitive to **animals** can experience contact H/S following animal exposure. The mechanism is probably mediated by IgE antibodies to animal proteins.

RECOMMENDATIONS:

Appropriate skin tests or IgE RAST tests to **animal** proteins.

#79. LATEX PROTEIN: Contact exposure to **latex protein** in gloves, balloons, condoms, and other products can cause contact H/S. This is considered an IgE antibody-mediated mechanism.

RECOMMENDATIONS:

IgE RAST test to **latex**. Unfortunately, there is no commercially available skin test for latex. The test must be prepared by a healthcare professional, usually an allergist.

#80. SKIN CONTACT WITH FOOD: Direct skin contact with **foods**, such as shellfish, fish, peanuts, etc. can cause H/S. I evaluated a young woman who had recurring H/S on the "V" area of her neck. She was wearing a necklace made of nuts from Hawaii. Careful examination of the necklace revealed small cracks in a few of the shells. A skin test made from the meat of the nut induced a positive test, proving that she had developed an immediate contact allergy to the Hawaiian nut. Contact food allergy is considered an IgE antibody-mediated mechanism.

RECOMMENDATIONS:

Appropriate skin tests or IgE RAST tests to a **food** allergen.

#81, #82. DRUGS OR CHEMICALS such as antibiotics and local anesthetics in hemorrhoid or sunburn preparations can cause contact H/S. In some cases, H/S are induced by an IgE antibody-mediated mechanism, while other drugs or chemicals may induce H/S through non-immune mechanisms (**chapter 1**).

RECOMMENDATIONS:

Refer to (**#50, chapter 5**).

#83. COSMETICS, HEALTHCARE PREPARATIONS. Shampoo and hair conditioner containing foreign animal proteins or nettle extract may cause contact H/S around the eyes, face and scalp. Oral preparations of bee pollen for hay fever treatment can cause contact H/S in the mouth and throat. Detergents may contain enzymes that may cause H/S and spot removers, fabric softeners, dryer sheets (static reducing laundry products) may contain perfumes that can cause contact allergic or contact photo-allergic H/S. H/S may result from IgE-mediated mechanisms or from non-immune mechanisms (**chapter 1**).

Recommendations:

Evaluation of **cosmetic and healthcare products** may include patch testing by applying diluted topical products onto aluminum discs called Finn Chambers. The chambers can be purchased at Allerderm Company (Petaluma CA, www.allerderm.com). It is advisable to dilute chemicals and products before patch testing to avoid severe irritant reactions. Allerderm can provide information on the appropriate dilutions for testing common topical healthcare products. A good reference for proper patch test dilution is listed in the reference section (DeGroot AC, 1994). Common patch test chemicals and allergens can be ordered from Allerderm Inc., for use with T.R.U.E. test kits (Petaluma CA). More unusual patch test chemicals can be ordered from Pharmascience Inc. (Montreal, Canada). A dermatologist or allergist can also provide guidance. Patch tests to these materials should be read at 30 minutes, 48 and 72 hours after application to detect immediate and delayed sensitivity reactions.

- There is one simple screening test that can be used to test cosmetics, lotions, shampoos and other healthcare products. Apply a single product behind one knee and on the flexion area of an elbow. The other untested side serves as a negative control. A healthcare professional should read the tested areas at 30 minutes, 48 hours, and 72 hours after application. A positive test may include any of the following: redness, itching, or wheal production. Use of the product should be discontinued if any of these responses occur.

#84 THROUGH #91A. HISTORY OF AUTOIMMUNE DISEASE: H/S has been described in association with **systemic autoimmune diseases** which may affect several organ systems. Refractory angioedema, with or without hives, has been reported as a manifestation of **systemic lupus erythematosus**. One recent report (Confino-Cohen, 2002) indicates some patients with chronic hives exhibit abnormal regulation of an immune pathway (p21 Ras) that is associated with systemic autoimmune diseases.

There are other examples of autoimmunity associated with H/S, such as the association with **autoimmune thyroiditis, (#54, #55, chapter 5).** In addition, recent studies have demonstrated a high prevalence of autoantibodies to IgE and to IgE receptors on mast cells in patients with chronic idiopathic urticaria (**chapter 1**).

Acquired angioedema in adults may be a manifestation of an autoimmune disorder caused by autoantibodies to C_1 esterase inhibitor.

It is not within the scope of this book to list every symptom or sign of autoimmune diseases. Nevertheless, individuals with H/S and multi-system symptoms may need an evaluation for systemic autoimmune disease.

GENERAL RECOMMENDATIONS:

The following screening tests should be ordered if an **autoimmune disorder** is suspected: CBC, ESR, chemistry screen, ANA and ENA profile, C_{1q}, autoantibody for C_1 esterase inhibitor, C_4, thyroid screen (free T_4, TSH, and perioxidase/thyroglobulin anti-thyroid antibodies).

- A screening test to assess the presence of **circulating auto-antibodies** in H/S can be assessed by the following method: a small volume (0.05ml) of serum from the patient is injected intradermally into the same individual. A control, using the same volume (0.05 ml) of normal saline, is also injected intradermally. A wheal and flare response within ten to thirty minutes in conjunction with a negative control suggests the presence of circulating autoantibodies against IgE or antibodies to IgE receptors located on mast cells. It is important to recognize that antihistamines can suppress this response; thus patients must not take these medications for a minimum of four days before this test is performed.

Confirmation tests using histamine release and in-vitro methods to detect the presence of circulating autoantibodies are not commercially available.

The demonstration of circulating autoantibodies can be useful as a therapeutic marker to justify use of steroids to treat the inflammation of chronic urticaria. Immunosuppressants, such as cyclophosphamide and cyclosporine (**chapter 7**), can decrease circulating autoantibody concentrations in these patients. Therefore, the demonstration of circulating autoantibodies may justify the use of immunosuppressants and/or steroids in these patients which predictably have more severe chronic urticaria.

- **Skin biopsies** of chronic urticaria characteristically reveal inflammation with perivascular cell infiltrates of monocytes, CD4+ lymphocytes, neutrophils, and eosinophils. The effects of mast cell degranulation initiated by autoantibodies and complement-activated products (C5a) are probably responsible for the inflammation seen in this disorder. Fluorescent antibody staining may be appropriate.

#84. JOINT INVOLVEMENT with H/S may suggest **rheumatoid arthritis, mixed connective disease, or systemic lupus erythematosus**. Bone X-rays, bone scan, ANA and ENA profiles, rheumatoid factor, and HLA tests would be appropriate.

#85. DRYNESS OF THE MOUTH OR EYES occurring with H/S may suggest **Sjogren's syndrome**, which would require testing for Sjogren's antibodies (anti-SSA or anti-SSB, also called anti-Ro or anti-La), and the measurement of tear volume.

#86. LUNG SYMPTOMS that accompany H/S may occur in systemic autoimmune disorders, such as **lupus** and **Sjogren's syndrome**. Evaluation could include ANA and ENA profiles, Sjogren's antibodies (anti-SSA or anti-SSB, also called anti-Ro or anti-La), tear volume, chest X-ray, and pulmonary lung functions.

#87. GASTROINTESTINAL SYMPTOMS occurring with H/S may suggest the need to evaluate for **inflammatory intestinal disease**, which at the minimum, would involve X-rays of the gastrointestinal tract and endoscopy.

#88. KIDNEY SYMPTOMS occurring with H/S may suggest the need to evaluate for autoimmune disease, such as **lupus erythematosus**. Evaluation may include ANA and ENA profiles, urinanalysis, urine culture, kidney function tests, such as creatinine clearance, BUN, skin biopsy and other appropriate tests.

#89. MUSCLE, SKIN AND NERVE SYMPTOMS occurring with H/S may require muscle and skin biopsies, ANA and ENA profiles, serum aldolase and creatine kinase levels, electromyography, skin biopsy, and other tests to rule out autoimmune diseases, such as **dermatomyositis (#28E, chapter 5)**.

#90. SKIN SYMPTOMS, such as sunlight sensitivity occurring with H/S, may suggest **lupus erythematosus.** The evaluation may require ANA and ENA profiles, skin biopsies for routine H&E stains, as well as immunofluorescence stains.

#91. THYROID EVALUATION FOR AUTOIMMUNE THYROIDITIS may require a thyroid screen (free T_4, TSH and perioxidase/ thyroglobulin anti-thyroid antibodies).

#91A. ACQUIRED ANGIOEDEMA without any recognizable cause should be evaluated for an underlying disorder with studies described in **#26E and #39, chapter 5**. Typically, C_4 and C_{1q} levels are decreased with acquired angioedema. Evaluation should also include testing for C_1 esterase inhibitor autoantibodies. ANA and ENA panels may also be appropriate. Some patients with C_1 esterase autoantibody may eventually develop a malignant lymphoproliferative disorder. Continued surveillance for this possibility is advised.

#92. HISTORY OF ANAPHYLACTIC SYMPTOMS ACCOMPANYING H/S. It is essential to determine whether anaphylactic symptoms accompany H/S, as patients with this complication may experience unconsciousness, shock and even death. Any or all of the symptoms listed in **#92** of the history questionnaire may suggest anaphylaxis is accompanying H/S. The cause of anaphylaxis may be idiopathic or associated with recognized causes. Detection and early treatment of this complication is essential.

Anaphylaxis can exhibit biphasic (two episodes separated by an asymptomatic interval of 1 to 8 hours), and protracted clinical patterns. Prolonged or recurrent episodes are more likely if the offending agent was taken orally or if the onset was 30 minutes or more after exposure to the anaphylactic stimulus. These observations underscore the need to follow patients carefully after an apparent remission of symptoms.

RECOMMENDATIONS:

A beta tryptase blood level should be obtained within **two hours** of the onset of symptoms if **anaphylaxis** is suspected with H/S. An elevated level can document an anaphylactic event.

Screening for allergens that may cause anaphylaxis would include RAST tests or skin puncture tests. Beta blockers can block adrenalin treatment of anaphylaxis. Consequently, beta blockers should be discontinued prior to skin testing.

#93. HISTORY OF H/S IN ASSOCIATION WITH SEXUAL INTERCOURSE, DURING OR UP TO 8 HOURS AFTER. H/S has been reported in association with intercourse. The temporal relationship is usually close to the time of intercourse, although delayed symptoms of H/S have been described up to 8 hours after intercourse. On occasion, symptoms of anaphylaxis may accompany H/S during intercourse.

Case reports (Didier EM, 1990) have described H/S during condom-protected sexual intercourse. The latex protein in condoms is considered a likely cause of this occurrence. There are also case reports (Green RL, 1985; Greenberger PA 1991) in which H/S developed following contact with antibiotics in coital secretions.

Contact with seminal fluid has induced immediate hypersensitivity reactions. Some persons may develop IgE antibodies to seminal fluid protein(s), causing H/S. Another report (Mike N, 1995) described a young woman who developed H/S with arthralgias approximately 8 hours after intercourse. The authors suggested immune complex formation as a possible mechanism.

RECOMMENDATIONS:

- A beta tryptase blood level should be obtained **within two hours** of onset of **anaphylactic** symptoms. An elevated level can document an anaphylactic event.

- Latex IgE RAST test would be appropriate if the history suggests **latex sensitivity** (**#43, chapter 5**)

- Evaluation for **drug sensitivity** would be a consideration if anaphylaxis occurs during sexual intercourse and the partner had been taking an antibiotic or other medication (**# 50, chapter 5**).

- Evaluation of **seminal fluid sensitivity** requires an IgE RAST to seminal fluid (available through Johns Hopkins Dermatology, Allergy and Clinical Immunology Reference Laboratory: Address P.O. Box 26037, Baltimore, MD 21224; Tel. 800-344-3224). Referral to an immunologist/allergist would also be appropriate.

#94. HISTORY OF SURGICAL OPERATION(S) WITHIN TWO YEARS PRIOR TO ONSET OF H/S.

The coexistence of H/S with a post-operative infection, such as a **draining bacterial wound at a surgical site**, should be evaluated. The case report in "**history of recent infection**" (**#58 in chapter 5**) underscores the possible relationship between chronic bacterial infections and H/S.

RECOMMENDATIONS:

- Evaluation of a **post-operative infection** may require CBC, ESR, chemistry screen, specific diagnostics (X-rays, cultures) and total complement CH_{50}.

- There is sparse literature suggesting **metal implants** may occasionally be associated with H/S. Some companies such as Medtronics, Inc. will supply component samples of implants for patch testing.

CHAPTER 6

TREATMENT
RECOMMENDATIONS

"Hives (urticaria) and/or swellings (angioedema)" are usually abbreviated as H/S in this chapter.

Citations for treatment are listed in the reference section under "Treatment". On occasion an important citation is noted in the text.

The purpose of this chapter is to outline a comprehensive plan for the management of H/S. The management of these conditions is divided into two parts.

PART A describes general management guidelines for H/S, regardless of cause. It includes:

- Treating the immediate H/S crises to control symptoms and prevent the development of systemic anaphylactic shock reactions.
- Avoiding non-specific factors that may intensify and worsen symptoms of H/S.
- Instituting general medical treatment to suppress on-going symptoms of H/S.

> **PART B** describes the treatment of specific causes of H/S. It includes:
> - Identifying the cause of H/S.
> - Initiating procedures to avoid specific triggers of H/S.
> - Treating a specific cause.

PART A:
GENERAL MANAGEMENT GUIDELINES
FOR H/S, REGARDLESS OF CAUSE

I. TREATMENT OF IMMEDIATE H/S

An acute episode of H/S may be a warning sign of systemic anaphylaxis. Patients may not recognize symptoms of anaphylaxis that can accompany H/S. Consequently, patients with acute onset of H/S should be evaluated in an office equipped to treat anaphylaxis. The management of acute H/S may involve the following approaches:

- Clinical assessment is advisable to detect symptoms or signs of anaphylaxis. Rapid heart rate, flushing, sweating, low blood pressure, dizziness, nausea or vomiting, metallic taste in the mouth, difficulty breathing, hoarseness, difficulty swallowing, decreased alertness and loss of consciousness may be indicators of anaphylaxis. A blood elevation of beta-tryptase can diagnose or confirm anaphylaxis. There is a **two-hour** interval from the time of onset of symptoms to detect elevations of beta tryptase.

- If the assessment suggests anaphylaxis, immediate steps should be initiated to reverse this complication:
  - Assessment of airway, breathing, and circulation.
  - Endotracheal intubation or cricothyrotomy, if needed.

- Place in recumbent position.
- Aqueous epinephrine intramuscular injection(s) into deltoid or anterolateral thigh. For adults, 1:1000, 0.3ml-.5 ml intramuscularly, as needed every 5-10 minutes, to control blood pressure and symptoms. For children, 0.01 mg/kg, up to a maximum dose of 0.3 mg. Side effects: rapid heart rate, headache, tremors.
- Administer oxygen, 6-8 L/min.
- Intravenous fluids (normal saline or plasma expanders, as needed).
- Systemic glucocorticosteroids (hydrocortisone, methylprednisolone) intravenously or orally. This is not usually helpful for the immediate situation, but may prevent prolonged anaphylaxis.
  - Initially side effects are minimal. However, side effects can occur if the patient remains on this medication for several months. The use of long-acting steroids, such as triamcinolone (Kenalog®) is contraindicated as this medication has a longer time of onset and persists in the body up to one month.
- Antihistamines by injection or orally. An H_1 antihistamine, such as diphenhydramine (Benadryl®), may be used. For adults, administer 50 mg every 6 hours orally, or by intravenous administration up to a maximum of 400 mg daily. For children, administer 1mg/kg every 6 hr up to a maximum of 300 mg per day. H_2 antihistamines, such as ranitidine (Zantac®), may also be administered with Benadryl. Ranitidine doses for adults are 50 mg intravenously or orally and may be repeated every 6 hours; for children, 1 mg/kg and repeat every 12 hours as needed.
- Nebulized albuterol and/or intravenous aminophylline (5 mg/kg) over 30 minutes for bronchospasm.
- Vasopressors to support low blood pressure, such as dopamine (400 mg in 500 ml of 5% dextrose in water, intravenously at 2-20 microgram/kg/min, titrating the rate to control blood pressure).
- Glucagon, if the patient is taking a beta blocker. Administer 1-5 mg (20-30 microgram per kg, to a maximum of 1 mg in children) intravenously over 5 minutes, followed by infusion of 5-15 micrograms/minute. Caution: may cause nausea and vomiting.

- Monitor for delayed recurrence of anaphylactic shock that may occur during the next 24 to 36 hours following onset of symptoms.
  - Continued oral or intravenous administration of cortisone and antihistamines may be required for 24 to 48 hours to prevent delayed recurrence of anaphylactic shock.
- It is advisable to prescribe a self-administered adrenalin kit (Epipen®) to patients who have experienced anaphylaxis with H/S.

II. Avoidance of non-specific factors that can intensify and worsen symptoms of H/S

H/S can be worsened by the following non-specific factors:

- Alcoholic beverages.

- Non-steroid anti-inflammatory medication such as:
  - Aspirin (AlkaSelzer®; Empirin®)
  - Ibuprofen (Motrin®; Advil®)
  - Naproxen (Naprosyn®)

- Codeine and other opiate medications used for pain control:
  - oxycodone (Percodan®; Percocet®); morphine (Avinza®); meperidine (Demerol®); pentazocine (Talwin®).

III. Institute general medical treatment to suppress symptoms of H/S, regardless of cause

There are some controversies associated with the general treatment of H/S, such as:

- Deciding which medications are the most suppressive with the least amount of side effects.

- Is it better to use one medication or a combination of medications to achieve the best results?

- Is it reasonable to prescribe medications at doses higher than approved by the FDA?

There are minimal studies that have compared the suppression of H/S using different antihistamines. Consequently, the recommendations in this section are not entirely based on evidence-based data, but may include the *"art of medicine"* observations compiled from my own experience, as well as from other clinicians.

It is important to have a realistic goal of symptom suppression. In my experience, this means achieving reduction of H/S while minimizing the side effects of medications. It does not always mean complete elimination of H/S, which may require higher doses of steroids and antihistamines.

Healthcare professionals frequently combine different categories of medications in an attempt to achieve optimal suppression of symptoms. The following outline lists the various therapeutic approaches commonly used to suppress H/S:

Treatment with H_1 blocker antihistamines (first, second, and third generation antihistamines):

First generation antihistamines **(FGAH)** refer to the first marketed drugs of that category and typically are associated with sedation. The second **(SGAH)** and third generation **(TGAH)** antihistamines are the more recently marketed antihistamines. They have minimal or no sedative side effects. FGAH, SGAH and TGAH are considered H_1 histamine receptor blockers and do not affect H_2 histamine receptors.

Most healthcare professionals use SGAH and TGAH as the initial medications to treat H/S. The goal of treatment of H/S with SGAH and TGAH is to control itching, and minimize recurring H/S. There are only a few studies that have compared the histamine (H_1) blocking activity of SGAHs. One study compared fexofenadine (Allegra®) and cetirizine (Zyrtec®), using standard approved daily doses. It appears that cetirizine has a longer duration of suppressive action (19 hours) compared to 9.3 hours for fexofenadine. Another study indicated that fexofenadine is a more potent H_1 blocker, compared to loratadine and chlorpheniramine. In a third study, fexofenadine exhibited faster onset and greater magnitude of wheal and flare suppression compared to desloratadine.

The available SGAH and TGAH are:

- Fexofenadine (Allegra®): The recommended dose for adults is 60 mg twice a day, and for children (ages 6-11 yr.), 30 mg twice a day. Studies suggest a dose of 120 mg twice a day for adults is more suppressive of symptoms. More recent studies indicate that doses in the range of 180 mg twice a day are well tolerated. Both 120 mg bid and 180 mg bid are off-label schedules. Side effects: none.

- Loratadine (Claritin®): The recommended dose for adults is 10 mg once a day, and for children (ages 2-5 yr.), 5 mg once a day. Side effects: none.

- Desloratadine (Clarinex®) is a TGAH: The recommended dose for adults and children (>12 yr) is 5 mg daily. Side effects: none.

- Cetirizine (Zyrtec®): The recommended dose for adults is 10 mg once a day, and for children (6 months to 6 years), 2.5 mg daily. The dose is 5-10 mg daily for older children (>6 yr.). This SGAH exhibits some anti-inflammatory effects involving eosinophils. Side effects: mild drowsiness in a small percentage of patients, but this can be minimized by taking it at bedtime.

SGAH and TGAH have been used in combinations of two, three or four medications. Obviously, a combination of more than two medications is very cumbersome and expensive for patients. Only a few studies have compared the suppressive effects of these medications, so the healthcare professional must experiment to determine which SGAH/TGAH or combination is more efficacious. What works for one patient may not be effective for another.

The **first generation antihistamines (FGAH)** are still commonly used to treat H/S. They are generally less expensive than SGAHs. As a group, they have become less popular in the treatment of H/S, because they cause significant sedation, especially at higher doses which may be needed to control symptoms. **Patients should be cautioned against driving, operating machinery or using tools while on these medications.** They may have insidious adverse effects on learning and academic performance in children. The goal of treatment of H/S with FGAH is to control itching and minimize the swelling and spreading of H/S. It is unusual to completely suppress H/S with a FGAH.

There are five classes of FGAHs. It is sometimes necessary to choose a FGAH from a different class in the event a FGAH is not effective or has serious side effects.

- Hydroxyzine (Atarax® and Vistaril®). The dose should be carefully titrated for adults and children. Adult doses begin at 10 mg to 20 mg at night, and then may be increased, depending on the severity of the H/S symptoms and the side effects, such as sedation. Children's doses start at 5-10 mg at night, depending on age and weight. Sedation can be mild to extreme, but patients adapt to this side effect. I *do not prescribe this medication for daytime consumption.* Avoidance of alcohol is also advised when taking this medication. Hydroxyzine can cause urinary retention in males who have enlargement of the prostate. This medication has been studied extensively and appears to be one of the more potent FGAHs for H/S treatment.

- Cyproheptadine (Periactin®) is a very potent FGAH that may also exhibit inhibitory effects against other mediators. The adult dose should be titrated, beginning with 4 mg at night, and gradually increased as needed. I *rarely prescribe this medication for daytime consumption because the main side effect is sedation.* Avoidance of alcohol is also advised when taking this medication. Cyproheptadine is associated with urinary retention in males who have enlargement of the prostate, and may increase pressure in the eye. It is associated with increased appetite and weight gain.

- Doxepin (Sinequan®) is a very interesting FGAH medication, as it exhibits both H_1 and H_2 antihistamine blocking properties. Dosing for adults begins at 10 mg to 20 mg at night and can be increased by 10 mg increments. This medication should be titrated carefully, as it causes sedation. I *prescribe it almost exclusively for nighttime consumption.* Patients should be informed in advance that this medication is primarily used as an anti-depressant; however it may be effective for treatment of H/S. Avoidance of alcohol is advised when taking this medication. Doxepin may cause blurred vision in glaucoma patients and urinary retention in males who have enlargement of the prostate.

Combinations of FGAH, SGAH and TGAH are often prescribed to treat H/S. A typical combination might include a SGAH during the daytime, which provides an antihistamine effect with minimal or no sedation, and a FGAH at night, which takes advantage of the sedative side effects of this group. The combination of cetirizine (Zyrtec®) with the FGAH hydroxyzine (Atarax® or Vistaril®) might produce unexpected side effects, since cetirizine is a metabolite of hydroxyzine. The combination can produce higher blood levels of cetirizine that may cause increased sedation.

The goal of treatment of H/S with SGAH, TGAH, and FGAH is to control itching, and minimize swelling and the recurrence of H/S. It is unusual to completely suppress H/S with these medications. *There have only been a few studies to determine whether combination treatment with FGAH and SGAH/TGAH is more efficacious than treatment with a single drug.*

It is sometimes helpful to perform a skin test (skin puncture method) to histamine with a saline control when treating with antihistamines. There may not be adequate histamine blockage if the histamine test produces a significant wheal and erythema response. In this event, it may be useful to increase antihistamine dosage(s) or to change antihistamines.

Combination of H_1 antihistamine receptor blockers (first, second and third generation antihistamines) with antihistamines that have H_2 blocking activity:

H_2 blocking antihistamines do not effectively control H/S. However, some clinicians believe that combining FGAH/SGAH H_1- and H_2-blocking antihistamines may be more effective in treating H/S than H_1-blocking antihistamines alone. *There is minimal data to support the belief that the combination of H_1- blocking antihistamines (FGAH and/or SGAH) and H_2-blocking antihistamines is more efficacious than treatment with H_1-blocking antihistamines alone.*

The commonly prescribed H_2-blocking antihistamines are:

- Cimetidine (Tagamet®); Ranitidine (Zantac®): These were developed for the reduction of stomach acidity, but may be used orally and/or intravenously to treat acute and chronic H/S. The adult dose for cimetidine is 200 mg to 400 mg (daily or bid) and 150 mg to 300 mg (daily or bid) for ranitidine. Side effects from these medications are rare, but may include headaches, muscle aches, dizziness, dry mouth, nausea, and fatigue.

- Doxepin (Sinequan®) is a very interesting FGAH medication as it blocks both H_1 and H_2 receptors. Consequently, its solitary use can sometimes answer the question of whether H_1- and H_2-blocking antihistamines might be helpful in treating H/S. This medication should be titrated carefully as it causes sedation. I *prescribe it almost exclusively for nighttime consumption.* The beginning dose for adults is 10 mg to 20 mg at night. The dose can be increased by 10 mg increments depending on clinical assessment. Patients should be informed in advance that this medication is primarily used as an antidepressant, but that it may be effective for treating H/S. Avoidance of alcohol is also advised when taking this medication. Doxepin may also cause urinary retention in males who have enlargement of the prostate and blurring of vision.

Anti-leukotrienes

I recommend reading **chapter 1** for an explanation of mediators and leukotrienes. Antihistamines cannot block the action of non-histamine mediators, such as **leukotrienes, chemokines, prostaglandins, platelet activating factor, bradykinin, etc**. The production and activity of leukotrienes can be blocked by available medications, such as, montelukast (Singulair®), zafirlukast (Accolate®), and zileuton (Zyflo®) which are referred to as **anti-leukotrienes**. A few evidence-based trials have established the effectiveness of these medications in the treatment of H/S. There is currently no FDA approval for treatment of H/S with anti-leukotrienes. Nevertheless, healthcare professionals do occasionally prescribe them as part of treatment regimens. *Although I do include them, I remain undecided as to the effectiveness of these medications.*

Sympathomimetics

Sympathomimetics, such as epinephrine and terbutaline can cause vasoconstriction which minimizes leakage of fluid through blood vessel walls, thereby inhibiting H/S formation. Terbutaline (Brethine®) is a beta$_2$ agonist that has fewer side effects on the heart and cardiovascular system compared to epinephrine. In general, epinephrine or terbutaline can be administered by injection to treat acute flare-ups of H/S. Oral terbutaline can be added to suppress recurring symptoms. Terbutaline can be associated with tremulousness and rapid heart rate, but these side effects can be reduced by titrating the dosage.

There is no FDA approval for treatment of H/S with terbutaline. However, healthcare professionals do occasionally prescribe it as part of treatment regimens. I *do not prescribe this medication for nighttime consumption as it can cause sleeplessness.*

Steroids

Adrenal glucocorticosteroids exhibit important physiological functions, such as anti-inflammatory effects, stress responses, electrolyte balance, calcium metabolism, blood pressure control, and carbohydrate metabolism. The normal physiological effects of adrenal steroids may transform into serious side effects when they are prescribed at high doses on a daily basis for several months. However, when used properly under close supervision, the benefits outweigh the risks and they will provide excellent control of H/S that are difficult to treat.

The goal of using steroids is to obtain optimal benefits with minimal side effects. This can best be accomplished by establishing a cooperative understanding between the healthcare professional and the patient. Patients need to understand that steroids cannot be taken without the supervision of a healthcare professional. A written plan should be provided to the patient which includes a dose schedule of steroids. The patient should be instructed to contact the healthcare professional weekly for dose adjustment. **I also require that patients sign an informed consent regarding the potential side effects of steroids.** I *do this because chronic H/S may require numerous steroid treatments intermittently and sometimes continuously over long periods of time.*

The following is a list of known side effects that may develop if patients remain on high doses of steroids for prolonged time periods:

- Mood swings.

- Increased appetite and weight gain.

- Acne.

- High blood pressure.

- Increased blood sugar.

- Osteoporosis with an increased tendency for bone fractures.

- Increased stomach acidity, ulcer flare-ups.

- Loss of blood supply to hips and other joints which may result in joint replacement.

- Increased eye pressure causing glaucoma.

- Cataract formation.

- Suppression of adrenal gland function. Patients on long-term steroids should inform their surgeons of this treatment, in the event surgery is contemplated.

The list of side effects is foreboding if taken out of context. In the hands of experienced healthcare professionals, the side effects may be diminished and prevented by carefully-controlled dosage of steroids. The most commonly prescribed steroid is prednisone, which can be taken orally once or twice a day in divided doses. Steroids should be reduced to a dose that maintains minimal suppression of symptoms and then switched to an every other day schedule to reduce side effects. As a general rule, one and one half times the suppressive dose can be taken the **on** day and nothing the **off** day. This dose can then be decreased slowly, as long as symptoms are controlled. As steroids are switched to doses every other day, other suppressive medications may be added or increased the **off** day of the steroid medication dose.

I prefer to use prednisone because it is eliminated from the body within 24 to 36 hours, thereby reducing the potential for side effects. Occasionally, some patients do not respond to prednisone. Empirically some of these patients respond better to methylprednisolone (Medrol®). There is no known medical reason to explain this observation, other than the speculation that prednisone needs to be metabolized to prednisolone by the liver in order to be pharmacologically active. Methylprednisolone is already in the active form.

Some healthcare professionals prescribe injectable steroids, such as intramuscular triamcinolone (Kenalog®) to control H/S. I do not recommend using injected triamcinolone because it remains in the body for periods of 30 to 45 days. This will cause prolonged suppression of the adrenal and pituitary glands and potentially more side effects.

My Treatment Regimen

I have outlined my treatment preferences for suppressing H/S with the following representations:

- My recommendations are based on a mix of evidence-based data and personal experience. I am not aware of scientific trials that have compared different treatment regimens for H/S. My recommendations are in italics to underscore the anecdotal nature of these recommendations.

- My recommendations have not been influenced by financial or business interests involving pharmaceutical companies.

- *I start patients on a second (SGAH) or third generation antihistamine (TGAH). I usually begin with fexofenadine (Allegra®) 120 mg (two 60 mg tablets) twice a day, or cetirizine (Zyrtec®), one 10 mg tablet at night. Desloratadine (Clarinex®) 5 mg daily is also an effective TGAH that may be used as the starting medication. Fexofenadine, cetirizine and desloratadine are interesting because they may have anti-inflammatory action, although these effects have primarily been demonstrated in animals or in vitro experiments. Nevertheless, an antihistamine with an anti-inflammatory effect could theoretically be more effective in suppressing H/S.*

- *I add a second SGAH or TGAH depending on the initial response.*

- *Topical application with 1% menthol in aqueous cream may be helpful in suppressing itching.*

- *If the patient has severe symptoms that cause functional impairment, I start prednisone 20 mg to 40 mg, twice a day.*

- *After one week on this regime, symptoms should be controlled sufficiently to begin reducing prednisone by 5 mg or 10 mg decrements every three days, with the goal of eliminating prednisone in two weeks, or beginning a dosage of prednisone every other day to minimize side effects. I switch to doses using one and one half the daily dose of prednisone for the day* **on** *treatment.*

- *I try to reduce the every other day dosage of prednisone by 5 mg or 10 mg decrements at least weekly. Sometimes the dose has to be reduced more slowly with 1 mg decrements.*

- In the event H/S symptoms increase the day **off** prednisone or during prednisone reduction, I consider:

  - Performing a skin puncture test with histamine and a saline control. If the histamine produces a significant wheal and flare, there is a good possibility histamine blockage is incomplete with oral antihistamines. In this case, I increase the antihistamine dosage.

  - I increase fexofenadine to 180 mg twice a day, especially the day **off** prednisone, and inform patients this dose is not approved by the FDA.

  - On the day the patient is **off** prednisone, I may also increase cetirizine to 10 mg twice a day, and inform patients they may experience sedation, as this is an off-label dose.

  - I may also add a first generation antihistamine (FGAH) at night, which is usually doxepin (Sinequan®), beginning with 10 mg to 20 mg, and depending on the severity of the symptoms, gradually increase this dose up to 50 mg to 60 mg as tolerated. An alternative FGAH that may be suppressive is cyproheptadine (Periactin®), beginning with 4 mg at night and if necessary increase by 4 mg increments up to 12 mg to 16 mg. These drugs produce significant sedation and cyproheptadine can increase appetite and cause weight gain. I choose these FGAHs because there is literature suggesting they may interfere in the biologic effects of histamine and other mediators that may cause H/S. Additionally, doxepin has antihistamine effects on both H_1 and H_2 receptors.

  - I may add a sympathomimetic, terbutaline (Brethine®), 10 mg in the morning and the afternoon.

  - I return to a daily regimen of prednisone if symptoms do not improve, or switch to methylprednisolone (Medrol®), using doses in the range of 8-12 mg, twice a day for adults. After one or two weeks, I try to reduce this dosage by 2-4 mg decrements every three days, or switch to an every other day schedule using one and one half the daily dose for the day **on** methylprednisolone.

  - I may add an anti-leukotriene (10 mg of Singulair®) to the regimen.

  - I may also add rofecoxib (Vioxx®) 25-50 mg Q.D. for a trial of one month to reduce production of other mediators (prostaglandin D_2 and leukotriene C_4).

  - Finally, if the H/S remain(s) unresponsive, I consider other therapies that are less conventional, less tried and associated with potentially more serious side effects. These treatments are described in **chapter 7**.

PART B:
MANAGEMENT OF SPECIFIC CAUSES OF HIVES (URTICARIA) AND/OR SWELLING (ANGIOEDEMA)

"Hives (urticaria) and/or swellings (angioedema)" are usually abbreviated as H/S.

I. ATTEMPT TO IDENTIFY THE CAUSE OF H/S

Assuming the immediate flare up is under control, the next effort should be to identify the cause of H/S. A method to achieve this goal is outlined in **Sections 2 and 3,** which encourages collaboration between the healthcare professional and the patient. Information obtained from the workbook, history questionnaire, physical examination, and results of laboratory tests are integrated to help identify possible cause(s) of H/S.

II. IF POSSIBLE, AVOIDANCE OF DEFINITIVE TRIGGERS OF H/S

Avoidance of a triggering factor that causes H/S is the ultimate method to control the recurrence of symptoms. In the example of acquired cold urticaria (**#32, Part B III, chapter 6**), avoidance of cold temperature conditions, such as swimming or skiing, would prevent the recurrence of symptoms. Similarly, individuals with sunlight-induced (solar) urticaria (**#31 Part B III, chapter 6**) should be able to minimize the recurrence of symptoms with sunscreens and by wearing clothing and hats that are impervious to ultraviolet rays. Other examples include avoidance of peanuts by patients with peanut allergy and exposure to latex products for latex-sensitive persons.

III. TREATMENT OF THE IDENTIFIED CAUSE OF H/S

Use the same number (#) from chapter 5 to find treatment recommendations for a specific cause of H/S. Please note that general suppressive treatment guidelines outlined in this chapter (Part A) may also be instituted to achieve more immediate control of H/S.

#1. HIVES, SWELLING, OR BOTH: Treatment should be tailored to the specific cause that may have been detected using the screening recommendations. Use the index to find the appropriate treatment section. In the event there is no specific diagnosis, refer to the general management guidelines in **chapter 6**, **part A**, and also to **chapter 7**, for guidelines on treating chronic H/S that are difficult to diagnose and treat.

#8,#9. FATIGUE; FEVER. There are multiple causes for these symptoms. Treatment recommendations should be targeted to a specific cause that has been confirmed by physical examination and laboratory tests. For example, the finding of a sore throat, enlarged lymph nodes and a positive blood test for mononucleosis would direct treatment to the management of infectious mononucleosis. The management of this condition might include: rest, symptomatic treatment of the sore throat and fever, and avoidance of contact sports to prevent potential injury to an enlarged spleen.

The presence of fever, eosinophilia, weight gain, recurring urticaria, and angioedema may suggest episodic angioedema with eosinophilia, which is self-limiting and responds to steroid therapy.

#10, #11. WEIGHT GAIN; WEIGHT LOSS: These symptoms are non-specific, but evaluation may lead to the confirmation of a diagnosis of hypothyroidism or hyperthyroidism with autoimmune thyroiditis and chronic H/S (**#54, #55, chapter 5**). Treatment recommendations for hypothyroidism may include careful thyroid hormone supplementation (**#54**), which over time, may lead to the resolution of the H/S. The finding of hyperthyroidism requires a consultation with an endocrinologist.

The presence of weight gain, fever, eosinophilia, recurring urticaria, and angioedema may suggest episodic angioedema with eosinophilia, which is self-limiting and responds to steroid therapy.

#12. EMOTIONAL SYMPTOMS: As part of a complete workup, the association of H/S with emotional symptoms (anxiety, depression, panic reactions or mood swings) may lead to the diagnosis of an unanticipated underlying medical disease. Treatment should be targeted at the underlying medical disease to determine whether it is causing the H/S and emotional symptoms.

The treatment of **adrenergic urticaria** will depend on the situations in which stress causes the hives. Avoidance of stressful conditions would be the simplest approach. If that is not practical, treatment with a beta-blocker such as propanolol, might effectively suppress symptoms. Counseling and the use of other pharmacological agents may also be required.

The treatment of **cholinergic urticaria** can be best controlled with H_1 antihistamines, hydroxyzine (Atarax®) and its metabolite, cetirizine (Zyrtec®).

#13. DRY SKIN: This symptom is non-specific, but the evaluation might lead to the confirmation of hypothyroidism with autoimmune thyroiditis and chronic H/S (**#54, chapter 6**). Treatment recommendations may include careful thyroid hormone supplementation which, over time, may lead to the resolution of the H/S.

#14. BRUISING EASILY: The causes of this symptom are multiple, but on rare occasions leukemia or urticarial vasculitis (**Appendix 1**) may cause H/S.

Immediate referral to a hematologist or oncologist is advised in the event leukemia or other cancerous condition is suspected or diagnosed.

Treatment of urticarial vasculitis requires a varied approach. Any combination of medications may be helpful in treating this condition, such as short courses of steroids, indomethacin, dapsone, colchicine, and hydroxychloroquine. A referral to an allergist, clinical immunologist or dermatologist may be appropriate if this disease is diagnosed. On occasion, urticarial vasculitis may be caused by an underlying disease, such as viral hepatitis, which if present, requires more specific treatment with alpha interferon, ribavirin and pegylated interferon. If viral hepatitis is diagnosed, a referral to a gastroenterologist or hepatologist is advised.

#15. HAIR LOSS: (#54, chapter 6)

#16,#17. TENDERNESS OVER FACE; DISCOLORED NASAL DRAINAGE: It may be advisable to treat sinusitis, tooth abscess, or gingivitis with appropriate antibiotics. Nasal steroids and decongestants would be advisable in the event sinusitis is diagnosed.

#18. PUFFINESS AROUND EYES: A diagnosis of **hypothyroidism with autoimmune thyroiditis** requires thyroid supplementation, **(#54, chapter 6)**

#19. SEVERE SORE THROAT; DIFFICULTY SWALLOWING; HOARSENESS: The diagnosis of an infectious disease causing a sore throat requires appropriate treatment.

The treatment of hoarseness or difficulty swallowing due to angioedema will depend on the underlying cause. General treatment would include the same recommendations for anaphylaxis described in **Part A, chapter 6**.

#20. COLD SORES: Recurring cold sores may be caused by Herpes Simplex virus. Treatment of this condition with anti-viral agents (acyclovir, Zovirax®; valacyclovir Valtrex®) is reasonable as this viral infection can cause a hive-like condition, namely erythema multiforme.

#21. TEETH ARE PAINFUL: Treatment of gingivitis, dental abscess, etc. requires referral to a dentist (**#16, #17, chapter 6**).

#22, #23. JOINT PAIN AND SWELLING: The diagnosis of an underlying autoimmune disease in association with H/S requires specific treatment of the autoimmune disease. A referral to a rheumatologist is advised. The use of steroids to treat H/S may suppress important clinical manifestations that are diagnostic of the underlying autoimmune disease. Hence, it may be advisable to defer use of steroids until a rheumatologist has evaluated the patient.

#23A. BONE PAIN: The cause of bone pain will determine the treatment approach. The treatment of **systemic mastocytosis** is discussed in **#29, chapter 6**. A diagnosis of **Schnitzler's syndrome** or **gammopathy** would require a referral to a hematologist or oncologist.

#24. MULTIPLE BONE FRACTURES: The recommended treatment for hyperparathyroidism is surgical removal of the parathyroid glands.

#25. CHRONIC COUGH, SHORTNESS OF BREATH, WHEEZING: It is not within the scope of this text to describe the treatment of all possible underlying pulmonary diseases. Treatment approaches are available through other resources, such as consultation with a pulmonologist or an allergist.

Episodic wheezing with H/S may be a manifestation of anaphylaxis that would require immediate treatment (**Part A, I, chapter 6**).

#26. GASTROINTESTINAL (GI) SYMPTOMS: It is not within the scope of this text to describe treatments for all potential underlying GI diseases. Treatment approaches are available through other resources, such as consultation with a gastroenterologist.

Episodic diarrhea, abdominal cramps and vomiting with H/S may be a manifestation of anaphylaxis that would require immediate treatment (**Part A, I, chapter 6**).

#26A. TREATMENT OF ANGIOEDEMA OF THE GASTROINTESTINAL TRACT CAUSED BY HEREDITARY OR ACQUIRED ANGIOEDEMA requires specialized therapies (**#39, chapter 6**).

#27. SYMPTOMS INVOLVING THE URINARY AND/OR REPRODUCTIVE SYSTEMS: It is not within the scope of this text to describe treatments for all potential underlying urinary and/or reproductive diseases. Treatment approaches are available through other resources, such as consultation with an appropriate specialist.

#28. SYMPTOMS OF MUSCLE AND/OR NERVE DISEASE: It is not within the scope of this text to describe treatments for all potential underlying neuro-muscular diseases. Treatment approaches are available through other resources, such as consultation with a neurologist.

Syncope with H/S may be a manifestation of anaphylaxis that would require immediate treatment (**Part A, I, chapter 6**).

#29. INDUCTION BY RUBBING OR SCRATCHING: Dermographism can be effectively suppressed with antihistamines. *Hydroxyzine (Atarax®; Vistaril®) and its metabolite cetirizine (Zyrtec®) are anecdotally reported to control dermographism. I prefer to start a low dose of hydroxyzine at night, and then gradually increase the dose to levels that suppress dermographism. The dose of hydroxyzine should be titrated with 10 mg increments and reduced if sedative side effects are significant. Patients should be cautioned about drinking alcohol while taking this medication. Cetirizine may be associated with mild sedation. I do not use hydroxyzine and cetirizine together, as the latter is the metabolite of hydroxyzine. Other antihistamines can also be tried, preferably the second-generation antihistamines. Steroids do not suppress dermographism.*

The late phase of biphasic dermographism is not responsive to antihistamines and may require low dose oral steroids on alternate days.

Patient education is helpful when treating this common condition. Awareness of the relationship between tight garments, scratching or rubbing and the induction of pruritic welts may help control symptoms and reduce the anxiety caused by experiencing these symptoms.

A diagnosis of **urticaria pigmentosa** or **mastocytosis** presents a more challenging treatment problem. There are no effective treatments for these conditions. Any of the first- or second-generation antihistamines can be added, but they usually do not completely suppress symptoms. Oral cromolyn is occasionally used to treat skin manifestations and diarrhea. Oral steroids do not alter these conditions, although there are some claims that topical steroids can reduce skin manifestations. A few studies claim improvement of symptoms with alpha-interferon.

All patients with mastocytosis should be prescribed an emergency adrenalin kit (i.e. Epipen), in the event they are exposed to situations that could lead to massive histamine release. Triggers of histamine release would include bee stings, extreme temperature changes, massage, ingestion of alcohol, X-ray procedures with radio-contrast media, and medications, such as opiates and dextran volume expanders. Additionally, patients with mastocytosis are prone to ulcers in the stomach and the upper intestinal tract. Consequently, it is advised that patients receive medications to reduce stomach acids, such as proton pump inhibitors, i. e. esomeprazole, (Nexium®); lansoprazole (Prevacid®); and H_2 antihistamines, i.e. cimetidine (Tagamet®); ranitidine (Zantac®). The treatment of these disorders may require referral to a clinical immunologist or dermatologist. Mastocytosis may transform into a malignant condition that requires referral to an oncologist.

#30. SUSTAINED PRESSURE CAUSING PAINFUL SWELLING: The treatment of this condition is quite challenging. Avoidance is not always possible as symptoms may occur from normal daily activities, such as walking, which may induce painful swelling of the feet. Antihistamines do not control the deep swelling characteristic of this condition. Occasionally, aspirin or other NSAIDS (non-steroid anti-inflammatory drugs), such as ibuprofen(Advil®), naproxen (Naprosyn®), or indomethacin (Indocin®), may control and prevent symptoms. Rofecoxib (Vioxx®), a selective inhibitor of cyclooxygenase-2, may be effective as it reduces other mediators, namely, prostaglandin D_2 and leukotriene C_4. Oral steroids are helpful in treating this condition, but it is important to cite the cautions advised in **chapter 6** if intermittent or long-term treatment is necessary. It is advisable to start with daily high doses of prednisone (20 mg to 40 mg) and then switch to an every other day schedule within ten days. There are some reports claiming benefits with sulfasalazine (Azulfidine®), colchicine, and dapsone. According to (Nettis E et al), patients with deep pressure urticaria may benefit therapeutically with the combination of montelukast (Singulair®) and loratadine (Claritin®).Occasionally, symptoms may improve after the elimination of a food that produces a positive delayed skin test result. I *have observed that an* NSAID *daily, in combination with prednisone on alternate days, is frequently effective in minimizing the symptoms of this condition.* Singulair® *with a* SGAH *has also been helpful in treating this disorder.*

#31. EXPOSURE TO SUNLIGHT: Wearing sunscreen and clothing impervious to UV radiation may reduce the symptoms of solar urticaria. There is no therapeutic approach specifically effective for this disorder. A referral to a dermatologist may be advisable to confirm the condition and to consider alternative therapeutic options available through that specialty.

#32. COLD EXPOSURE: The primary objective of acquired **cold urticaria** management is the prevention of shock during exposure to cold water or other cold temperature conditions. Cold-induced shock during water activities may be associated with drowning. All cold urticaria patients are at risk of experiencing cold-induced shock reactions during water sports activities, regardless of whether a positive cold test can be elicited. Therefore, cold urticaria patients should avoid water sports activities until their symptoms have spontaneously resolved.

Management with medications has generally been very effective in suppressing the symptoms of acquired cold urticaria. There are well-controlled studies that have proven the efficacy of first-generation antihistamines (FGAH), such as cyproheptadine (Periactin®), doxepin (Sinequan®), hydroxyzine (Atarax®;Vistaril®) with cimetidine (Tagamet®),and ketotifin (not available in the United States). In addition, some data indicates beneficial suppression with second-generation antihistamines (SGAH). All of these medications may suppress the cold stimulation time test (**CSTT; #32, chapter 5).** When treating with a FGAH/SGAH, it is advisable to titrate with a low dose at night and gradually increase the dose until the CSTT is increased to more than three minutes, a time that correlates clinically with a lower percentage of cold-induced shock reactions. Oral steroids do not suppress the symptoms of cold urticaria.

It is important to treat underlying disorders that may cause cold urticaria, such as **chronic lymphocytic leukemia** or **cryoglobulinemia**, (**#32, chapter 5**). Referral to an oncologist would be appropriate. The association of **urticarial vasculitis** with **cold urticaria**, (**#32, chapter 5**) may require treatment with oral steroids.

Unpublished studies by Hal Hoffman, M.D. (hahoffman@ucsd.edu) suggest that a recombinant human interleukin-1 receptor antagonist (anakinra; Kineret®) may prevent symptoms of **familial cold auto-inflammatory syndrome**. Referral to an immunologist would be appropriate.

I prescribe an adrenalin kit (Epipen®) for all acquired cold urticaria patients, especially if they pursue water sports activities or are exposed to outdoor cold temperatures. Patients who pursue outdoor activities at cold temperatures, or swimming should, at the minimum, be prescribed suppressive FGAH or SGAH and perform these activities in the company of another individual.

#33. EXERCISE: There is no effective therapy to absolutely prevent **exercise-induced anaphylaxis**. There are, however, some recommendations that may reduce the likelihood of these events. Avoidance of triggers that may precipitate this condition is advisable, such as foods that have been identified by history or skin and/or IgE RAST tests. In general, patients should avoid exercise or even mildly strenuous activities, such as walking for two to four hours after eating. The patient should stop physical activity if any anaphylactic symptoms develop, such as H/S, flushing, or a sensation of fainting. Patients sensitive to airborne pollens should avoid exercise on days of high pollen counts. The prophylactic use of antihistamines may be of some benefit. Patients are advised to carry an adrenalin kit (Epipen®), wear a medical identification bracelet, and always exercise with another person. The ingestion of 1 tsp of sodium bicarbonate (baking soda) immediately before exercise may prevent these symptoms.

Cholinergic urticaria may be suppressed with hydroxyzine (Atarax®;Vistaril®). Some studies suggest prophylactic treatment with ceterizine may be beneficial for severe cholinergic urticaria. *Additionally, higher doses of ceterizine (10 mg bid), which are off-label, may control severe symptoms.*

#34. BATHING OR SHOWERING IN WARM TO HOT WATER: Heat-induced urticaria can often be controlled with prophylactic treatment using first- generation antihistamines (FGAH), particularly hydroxyzine (Atarax®; Vistaril®). The dosage should be titrated beginning at a low dose of 10-25 mg, at night.

I would recommend trials with SGAH before switching to FGAH.

#35. H/S FROM CONTACT WITH WATER, REGARDLESS OF TEMPERATURE: Aquagenic urticaria may be controlled with prophylactic treatment using first-generation antihistamines (FGAH), particularly hydroxyzine (Atarax®;Vistaril®). The dosage should be titrated, beginning at a low dose of 10-25 mg, at night.

I would recommend trials with SGAH before switching to FGAH.

#36 THROUGH #39. FAMILY HISTORY OF H/S: Except for the avoidance of triggering factors, there are no definitive treatments for the following hereditary syndromes: **vibratory angioedema (#36), familial dermographism (#29, chapter 6), familial exercise-induced anaphylaxis (#33, chapter 6), delayed cold urticaria**

(#32, chapter 6), familial aquagenic urticaria (#35, chapter 6). Treatment of familial cold auto-inflammatory syndrome is discussed in #32, chapter 6.

#39. HEREDITARY ANGIOEDEMA may be treated with prophylactic anabolic steroids, i.e. danazol (Danocrine®); stanazol, (Winstrol®) to prevent recurrent episodes. Short-term anabolic steroids, taken 4-5 days prior to elective dental or surgical procedures, may prevent angioedema. Liver functions should be monitored during treatment with anabolic steroids. Plasma concentrates of C_1 esterase inhibitor and fresh frozen plasma are available on an experimental basis to treat and prevent acute episodes of angioedema. Patients with this condition should be monitored with repeat C_4 levels. Persistently low levels may be an indication for prophylaxis with anabolic steroids.

C_{1q} levels are low in the acquired type of angioedema and should be monitored during remission. Anabolic steroids are helpful in treating this type of angioedema. Efforts should continue to recognize and treat the underlying cause of acquired angioedema.

Referral to an academic university center, allergist or clinical immunologist is advisable for hereditary and acquired angioedema.

#40. MUCKLE-WELLS SYNDROME can be treated with recombinant human interleukin-1 receptor antagonist (anakinra; Kineret®).

#41. HEREDITARY FEMALE HORMONE-DEPENDENT ANGIOEDEMA: There is no treatment other than discontinuation of estrogen supplementation, birth control medications, and recognizing the relationship of angioedema with pregnancy.

#42 THROUGH#49: OCCUPATIONAL HISTORY; HOME HISTORY; RECREATIONAL HISTORY

#42. HEALTHCARE OCCUPATION: The treatment of healthcare-related H/S depends on the cause of the condition. Occupational-acquired infectious illness will require specific treatments prescribed by a healthcare professional or an infectious disease specialist.

#43. LATEX SENSITIVITY: Latex sensitivity management requires avoidance of all latex products, and elimination of cross-sensitizing foods, such as avocados, bananas, kiwi, chestnuts, figs, melon, pineapple, peach, grapes, oranges and buckwheat. It may also be advisable to avoid application of skin creams and lotions that contain cross-reacting foods, such as avocado, banana, kiwi and watermelon. There is no therapy that can eliminate latex allergy.

Avoidance of latex requires diligence on the part of patients who need to be aware that it may be present in many commercial products, such as hair bonding glue, carpet padding, condoms, balloons and pacifiers. The American Latex Allergy Association (A.L.E.R.T) at www.latexallergyresource.org is an excellent site to learn about latex allergy.

#44,#45. ANIMAL EXPOSURE: Persons who are sensitive to animals should ideally avoid animal contact. However, avoidance of animals may be difficult when a person's livelihood is dependent upon animal care, such as veterinarians, veterinarian technicians and animal pet store personnel. Initiation of animal antigen immunotherapy may be indicated in those circumstances. Except for cat immunotherapy, supportive evidence remains sparse for immunotherapy for other animals.

#46. ARTS AND CRAFT SENSITIVITY: Avoidance is the mainstay for management of arts and craft induction of H/S.

#47. WATER ACTIVITIES OR COLD EXPOSURE: (#32, #34, #35, chapter 6).

#48. EXERCISE: (#33, chapter 6).

#49. WEIGHT-LIFTING: (#30, chapter 6).

#50. MEDICATION HISTORY: The mainstay of treatment is the elimination of medications or healthcare products that may cause H/S. When drug-induced H/S is a consideration, a withdrawal of all medications for 3 to 5 days may be necessary. Obviously, this may be difficult to do when patients are on essential medications.

On rare occasions, desensitization (a method of achieving tolerance to a medication by rapidly administering graduated doses of the medication orally or by injection), may be required to achieve tolerance to an essential medication, such as an antibiotic needed for the treatment of a life-threatening systemic infection.

Intravenous drug sensitivity to radiocontrast media can be minimized by 48 hour pre-treatment with oral steroids and antihistamines. Non-ionic radiocontrast media are associated with a lower incidence of H/S.

Herbal supplements are occasionally associated with rashes that may be confused as H/S. A classic example is a characteristic red rash (erythroderma) associated with St John's Wort which is used for the treatment of depression.

H/S or similar appearing rashes can occur in persons who have infectious mononucleosis while receiving certain antibiotics (ampicillin or levofloxacin).

Studies now indicate that specific COX-2 inhibitors can be used cautiously in patients with chronic H/S and aspirin sensitivity. Rofecoxib (Vioxx®) has a low incidence of cutaneous reactions in patients with asthma who have NSAID sensitivity (Stevenson DD, 2001).

ACE-Inhibitor induced angioedema can be a particularly difficult management problem that may be refractory to corticosteroids, H_1 and H_2 antihistamines, and epinephrine. In addition to discontinuing the causative ACE-Inhibitor, it may be necessary to treat with fresh frozen plasma (Karim et al) to reduce bradykinin levels that are implicated in causing the angioedema.

On occasion, H/S may persist weeks or months after a medication has been discontinued. The general explanation for this phenomenon is that some medications have long half-lives.

#51. INSECT HISTORY: Bee venom immunotherapy can reduce recurrence of H/S and systemic allergic reactions to repeat stings. The supporting studies have been demonstrated for yellow jacket, hornet, wasp, honeybee, and fire ant.

#52. FOOD HISTORY: The mainstay of treatment is the elimination of food or food additive exposure that can cause H/S. Studies now suggest that food sensitization can occur by routes other than oral ingestion. A study (Lack G et al 2003) showed that mothers who used creams containing peanut oil on their breasts while nursing may have sensitized their infants to peanut.

Healthcare professionals should consult patients about potential sensitivity to foods that are seemingly unrelated. For example, persons allergic to peaches are at high risk to develop allergic reactions to apricots, cherries and plums. Additionally, a person allergic to one tree nut such as peanut has an estimated risk of 40% to develop allergic reactions to other tree nuts. Complicating matters is the observation that persons with inhalant allergies to certain pollens, such as birch, can be unknowingly allergic to apples, celery, hazelnut, cherries and plums. A referral to a qualified allergist can be helpful in learning about cross reacting foods.

There is no scientifically established treatment that can improve tolerance to a food, such as "oral food drops" or crude food allergen injections. However, there is an important development on the horizon for patients with peanut allergy. A new humanized monoclonal anti-IgE antibody treatment is showing promise as a potential method to achieve tolerance to peanuts. Recent studies (Lueng D et al, 2003) indicate that administration of this vaccine increases the threshold of peanut protein required to induce allergic reactions. It could potentially eliminate life-threatening allergic reactions caused by inadvertent ingestion of small amouts of peanut. Unfortunately, it will be several years before it is approved by the FDA.

There is data (Vadas P et al) suggesting that peanut protein can be bound by activated charcoal. It is estimated that 40 mL of activated charcoal suspension (200 mg/mL) would be required to effectively complex the protein in one peanut. Hence, administration of activated charcoal may be a useful adjunct in treating small amounts of peanut antigen that has been accidentally ingested.

#53: TRAVEL HISTORY: The management of travel-related H/S is obviously dependent on the causative factor, such as identification of a specific infectious illness. Consequently, diagnosis and treatment are complementary because a specific infectious illness must first be identified and then treated in accordance with standard infectious disease treatment protocols.

#54 THROUGH #57. HORMONE HISTORY: The following hormone-related disorders associated with H/S include:

#54,#55. DISORDERS OF THE THYROID GLAND: Treatment of hypothyroidism or hyperthyroidism with autoimmune thyroiditis is indicated. On occasion, some individuals with H/S have normal thyroid hormone levels with evidence of autoimmune thyroiditis. It is possible H/S may resolve with small incremental supplements of thyroid hormone, even though thyroid levels are normal.

Autoimmune thyroiditis is caused by autoantibodies to thyroid antigens. One theory that may explain the association of urticaria and angioedema with autoimmune thyroiditis is the theory of molecular mimicry, which suggests there is molecular homology between thyroid autoantibodies and IgE receptors on mast cells. The addition of supplemental thyroid hormone might bind some of the circulating thyroid autoantibodies and thereby reduce the availability of these antibodies for attachment to IgE receptors on mast cells. Although hypothetical, it helps rationalize treatment of euthyroid H/S patients with thyroid hormone.

#56. OVERACTIVITY OF THE PARATHYROID GLAND: (#24, chapter 6).

#57. H/S COINCIDING WITH MENSTRUAL CYCLES: In this syndrome there is presumed to be auto-sensitivity to endogenous progesterone. The addition of birth control medications with little or no progesterone may be helpful in controlling symptoms. Additionally, there are case reports of progesterone sensitivity (listed in the references) which are controlled with anovulatory agents, such as LH-RH agonist (leuprolide acetate) and/or hysterectomy with bilateral salpingo-oophorectomy.

#57A. H/S COINCIDING WITH MENSTRUAL CYCLES: This syndrome appears to be caused by a decrease in progesterone levels. Treatment with oral medroxyprogesterone may control symptoms.

#57B. HEREDITARY ESTROGEN-DEPENDENT ANGIOEDEMA: There is no known treatment for this hereditary syndrome, other than discontinuing estrogen supplementation, birth control medications and avoiding pregnancy.

#57C. PRURITIC URTICARIAL PAPULES AND PLAQUES OF PREGNANCY (PUPPP): There are anecdotal reports suggesting oral steroids may be helpful in treating this syndrome. The use of oral steroids in pregnancy will require advice from an obstetrician.

#58 THROUGH #75. HISTORY OF RECENT INFECTION OCCURRING WITH H/S: The diagnosis and treatment are complementary as a specific infectious illness must first be identified and then treated in accordance with standard infectious disease treatment protocols. A referral to a specialist, such as an internist, pediatrician or an infectious disease specialist may be advisable.

#58A. FEVER: More common causes of fever need to be addressed and treated, depending on etiology. The presence of fever, eosinophilia, weight gain, recurring urticaria, and angioedema may suggest episodic angioedema with eosinophilia, which is self-limiting and responds to steroid therapy. Hereditary periodic fevers with H/S should be treated per diagnosis (**#32, #36 to #39, chapter 6**).

#58B. IMMUNE DEFICIENCY DISORDER: A diagnosis of symptomatic common variable immunodeficiency (CVID) may warrant treatment with intravenous immunoglobulin.

#76. HISTORY OF TUMORS, CANCERS WITH H/S: The diagnosis and treatment are complementary because a specific cancer or tumor must first be identified and then treated in accordance with standard cancer or tumor treatment protocols. A referral to a specialist, such as an internist, pediatrician, or an oncologist may be advisable.

The possibility of an occult lymphoma must be considered for patients with **acquired angioedema** and decreased C_{1q} levels. In this case, C_{1q} levels may be useful to monitor the presence or recurrence of a lymphoma.

#77 THROUGH #83. HISTORY OF ENVIRONMENTAL EXPOSURE THROUGH DIRECT SKIN CONTACT: The management of environmentally-induced contact H/S is primarily avoidance of suspect contact allergens.

It may be advisable to eliminate spot removers, fabric softeners, dryer sheets (static reducing laundry products) that may contain perfumes and detergents with enzymes. One detergent, "All Clear", does not contain these ingredients.

#84 THROUGH #91A: HISTORY OF AUTOIMMUNE DISEASE WITH H/S: The diagnosis and treatment are complementary because a specific autoimmune disorder must first be identified and then treated in accordance with standard rheumatology and immunology protocols. A referral to a specialist, such as an internist, pediatrician or a clinical immunology/rheumatology specialist may be advisable.

There is no recommended treatment for **autoantibodies that have specificity for IgE** or **IgE receptors on mast cells** other than utilizing the general management guidelines described in **chapter 6**. Reduction of these autoantibody titers has been achieved with immunosuppressant medications **(chapter 7)**.

Skin biopsies of chronic urticaria characteristically reveal inflammation with perivascular cell infiltrates of monocytes, CD4+ lymphocytes, neutrophils, and eosinophils. The effects of mast cell degranulation initiated by circulating autoantibodies and complement-activated products (C5a) are probably responsible for the inflammation seen in this disorder. The demonstration of circulating autoantibodies, using the test described in chapter 5, may be useful as a therapeutic marker to justify use of steroids to treat the inflammation of chronic urticaria.

#91. TREATMENT OF AUTOIMMUNE THYROIDITIS WITH H/S (#54, 55, chapter 6).

#91A. TREATMENT OF ACQUIRED ANGIOEDEMA (#39, chapter 6).

#92: HISTORY OF ANAPHYLACTIC SYMPTOMS ACCOMPANYING H/S: Treatment guidelines for anaphylaxis have been outlined in **Part A, chapter 6** and should be instituted to achieve control of H/S and anaphylaxis.

#93: HISTORY OF H/S ASSOCIATED WITH SEXUAL INTERCOURSE, DURING OR UP TO 8 HOURS AFTER. Treatment depends on the possible cause of these symptoms.

If the evaluation suggests **latex sensitivity** to condoms, avoidance of latex condoms and other latex products should be advised. In addition, avoidance of cross-reactive foods listed in **#43, chapter 6** would also be recommended.

The presumption of **allergic sensitivity to an antibiotic or drug** present in coital secretions would require avoidance of intercourse when a partner is taking these medications. Alternatively, the partner might use a protective barrier, although there is still a possibility for contact with coital secretions.

The possibility of an immunological **sensitivity to a protein in seminal secretions** must be considered. If this is established, the partner should wear a condom or avoid intercourse. Some allergists have performed immunotherapy with purified fractions of seminal fluid, but this approach is considered experimental.

#94. HISTORY OF SURGICAL OPERATION(S) WITHIN TWO YEARS PRIOR TO THE ONSET OF H/S. The diagnosis and treatment are complementary because a specific post-operative infection must first be identified and then treated in accordance with standard infectious disease treatment protocols. A referral to a specialist, such as a surgeon, internist, pediatrician, or an infectious disease specialist may be advisable.

The association of H/S with a surgical implant is not well-documented in the medical literature. Removal of an implant would not be considered a therapeutic solution unless definitive evidence for a cause and effect relationship can be established.

CHAPTER 7

CHRONIC HIVES AND/OR SWELLING WHICH ARE DIFFICULT TO DIAGNOSE AND TREAT

Hives (urticaria) and/or swellings (angioedema) are usually abbreviated as H/S.

Citations for treatment are listed in the reference section under "Treatment". An occasional citation is listed in the text.

Despite all best efforts, many patients are frustrated because their H/S cannot be diagnosed or treated effectively. It is incumbent to minimize patient concerns when they are told "there is nothing more that can be done". To overcome these concerns, the HCP should remain involved by encouraging continued re-evaluation of the clinical problem. It may be necessary to repeat the same process as before, namely the history, physical examination and certain laboratory tests. Sometimes the patient may recall an important fact while re-thinking the history. For example, one of my patients had a history of recurring H/S that implicated exercise as a potential cause. He forgot to mention that he was treated with sulfa for prostatitis a few weeks after his latest outbreak. This information provided a new explanation for his most recent exacerbation of H/S.

Repeating the process can also provide new observations that may lead to a definitive diagnosis. One of my patients with chronic H/S developed puffiness around her eyes and was eventually diagnosed with H/S secondary to autoimmune thyroiditis. The H/S eventually responded to thyroid medication.

A skin biopsy should be obtained in cases of hives that are difficult to diagnose and treat. Skin biopsies of chronic urticaria characteristically reveal inflammation with perivascular cell infiltrates of monocytes, CD4+ lymphocytes, neutrophils, and eosinophils. Two groups of chronic urticaria have been defined by skin biopsy results (Tharp MD, 1996): (1) perivascular lymphocyte predominant urticaria (PLPU), and (2) perivascular polymorphonuclear predominant urticaria (PPPU). Patients with PLPU are more responsive to antihistamines, while PPPU is more resistant to antihistamines and may require steroid treatment. The skin biopsy may also detect unsuspected urticarial vasculitis or mastocytosis. The latter requires metachromatic stains, such as Giemsa or Toluidine blue, for the detection of increased numbers of mast cells (usually >4 per high power field).

I also advise patients to keep daily diaries (**APPENDIX 2)**. Some physicians disapprove of this process because they believe that patients may develop an unhealthy obsession with their H/S. I believe the obsession does not have to be unhealthy if it focuses attention to details that may lead to uncovering the cause of symptoms. This process occasionally provides clues to diagnosis that were missed.

Finally, because of new knowledge about chronic H/S, I recommend that undiagnosed patients be tested for autoimmune antibodies that may be causing their symptoms. A screening test for the presence of circulating autoantibodies in chronic hive patients can be assessed by the following method: Collect serum from the patient. A small volume (0.05ml) of patient's serum is injected intradermally back into the same patient. A control using .05 ml of normal saline is also injected intradermally. An immediate wheal and flare response within 10 to 30 minutes in combination with a negative control suggests the presence of circulating autoantibodies to IgE receptors on mast cells. It is important to recognize that antihistamines can suppress this response; therefore patients must not take these medications for a minimum of four days before the test is performed. Confirmation tests using histamine release and in-vitro tests to detect the presence of autoantibodies are not commercially available.

The effects of mast cell degranulation initiated by circulating autoantibodies and complement-activated products (C5a) are probably responsible for the inflammation in this disorder. The demonstration of circulating autoantibodies may be useful as a therapeutic marker to justify use of steroids to treat the inflammation of chronic urticaria. In addition, immunosuppressants, such as cyclophosphamide, cyclosporine and tacrolimus (**chapter 7**), can decrease levels of circulating autoantibodies in these patients. Hence, the demonstration of circulating autoantibodies may help justify the use of these medications.

There are a number of therapeutic strategies that can be pursued for undiagnosed H/S. Unfortunately, the studies supporting these therapies are based on trials of small numbers of patients or single case reports. More importantly, these therapeutic strategies can be associated with some serious side effects. Overall, I do not suggest entering this realm of treatment options unless the patient is truly unresponsive to general treatment strategies **(chapter 6)**. It is unusual to achieve complete remission of symptoms. A realistic goal is reduction of symptoms that allow patients to return to normal daily activities.

The following treatment modalities have been used in small patient trials and are reported to improve refractory H/S. Please refer to reference section for citations under "**treatment**":

- **Cyclophosphamide (Cytoxan®)**: This is a potent immunosuppressant medication that has been used in severe unresponsive chronic H/S. A supportive case report (Bernstein et al, 2002) claims to have achieved clinical remission after 20 years of symptoms. The patient received intravenous doses of 500 mg followed by increases of 100 mg every 2 weeks. The maximum dose was 1,500 mg once a month. Coincidentally circulating autoantibodies were no longer detectable in this patient. Recommended PDR dosing is 1.5-3 mg/kg orally, daily. The side effects are multiple and may include effects on the liver, heart, kidney, bladder and bone marrow. Potential side effects should be carefully explained before use. It is advisable to involve an oncologist when prescribing this medication.

- **Cyclosporine (Neoral®)**: This is a potent immunosuppressant, although it works at a different level in the immune system than cyclophosphamide. Its effectiveness has been reported in a few case reports (listed in the reference section). One report claims a 50% improvement/resolution using 4 mg/kg dose daily. Side effects may involve the hepatic, renal and blood pressure systems. It is advisable to involve an oncologist when prescribing this medication. Blood levels of cyclosporine should be monitored to prevent toxic effects.

- **Tacrolimus (Prograf®)**: This immunosuppressant has been used in refractory H/S. It prevents mast cell and basophil cell degranulation and may have an inhibitory effect on cytokine expression. Dosing is 0.1 mg/kg orally every 12 hours. The dose is started at low levels and gradually increased depending on the response. Blood concentrations should not exceed 5-20 ug/ml. Renal, hepatic and blood pressure monitoring is advised. It is also advisable to involve an oncologist when prescribing this medication.

- **Dapsone**: This anti-leprosy medication has been shown to reduce H/S in a few patients. The side effects are primarily hematologic and hepatic. Close monitoring of CBC and liver functions is advised.

- **Fluoxetine (Prozac®)**: This selective serotonin reuptake inhibitor has been used successfully in the treatment of a single patient (Gupta MA, 1995) with refractory chronic idiopathic urticaria.

- **Methotrexate**: This immunosuppressant has also been used in uncontrolled small populations of H/S patients.

- **Sulfasalazine:** In one study, protracted treatment (6-8 weeks) with this antibiotic was reported to improve refractory H/S in 50% of the patients studied.

- **Plasmapheresis**: Apheresis is the process of collecting and separating blood components by automated cell separation equipment. Plasmapheresis is a type of apheresis sometimes used to remove harmful substances in the blood plasma of patients. This therapy is occasionally used to treat severe cases of H/S that do not respond to conventional therapies. Current thinking is that plasmapheresis removes circulating autoimmune antibodies to IgE or to IgE receptors on mast cells that may be responsible for chronic unremitting H/S.

Although effective, it is very costly and the benefits are not permanent as autoantibodies may recur.

- **Intravenous immunoglobulin**: Very limited reports suggest this therapy may be effective in select patients with circulating autoantibodies. There is some evidence that intravenous immunoglobulin may have an anti-inflammatory potential which may control autoantibody-mediated inflammation.

- **Acyclovir**: In one study of idiopathic chronic urticaria, 5 of 12 patients showed complete remission of symptoms with this medication. Discontinuation of acyclovir resulted in the reappearance of symptoms. The authors note these patients had high antibody titers to either Herpes Simplex or Epstein-Barr viruses, and conclude this medication produced its therapeutic effect by suppressing circulating viral antigen.

- **Rofecoxib (Vioxx®):** A recent study (Anand et al) described remission of idiopathic chronic urticaria in 5 of 8 patients treated with a COX-2 inhibitor, i.e. rofecoxib (Vioxx®) 25-50 mg qd. Theoretical rationale for using this medication is to reduce production of prostaglandin D_2 and leukotriene C_4, which can cause wheal and flare reactions. Patients with renal dysfunction should be excluded from treatment with this medication.

The future is hopeful for patients with undiagnosed, difficult-to-treat H/S, as new immunological and pharmacological therapies are developed. Successful treatment of H/S may eventually develop from the evolution of new antibody strategies, such as humanized, monoclonal anti-IgE antibody treatment for individuals with peanut allergy. Additionally, other novel vaccine approaches and innovative anti-mediator medications may bring therapeutic benefits for H/S patients. I believe these advances will eventually provide the medical profession with the tools to treat patients who suffer with the mystery and misery of these disorders

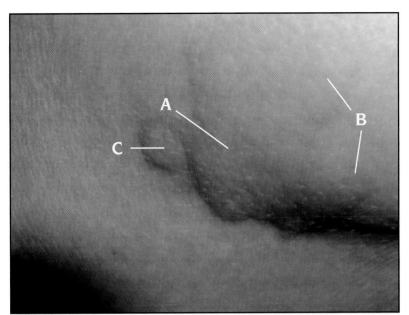

Figure 1: Hives (Urticaria) involving the right side of jaw with (A) raised pale, pink central area called a wheal or welt; (B) reddened border surrounding the central wheal and (C) satellite wheals.

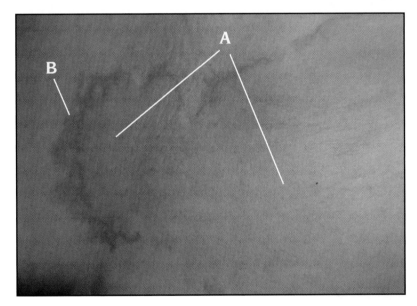

Figure 2: Giant Hives (Urticaria) involving the upper chest. (A) The wheal occupies a much larger area, sometimes the size of a grapefruit or larger. (B) Reddened border.

Figure 3: Swelling (angioedema) (A) involving entire upper lip, probably due to ibuprofen sensitivity.

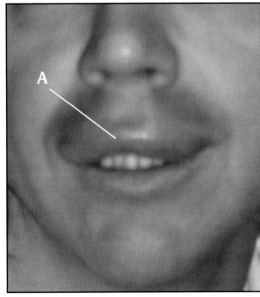

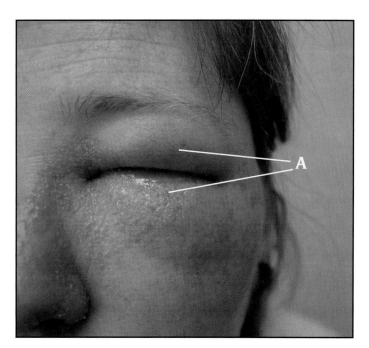

Figure 4: Swelling (Angioedema) involving the upper and lower eyelids due to an allergic reaction to ingested hazelnuts. (A) The swelling is more often one-sided, and in this example involves the left eyelids.

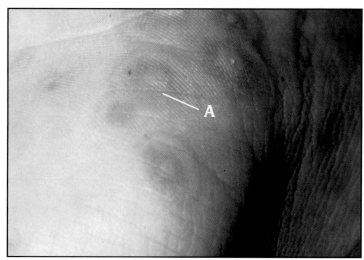

Figure 5: Erythema multiforme involving the palms. (A) The rash is raised and has a bull's eye target appearance.

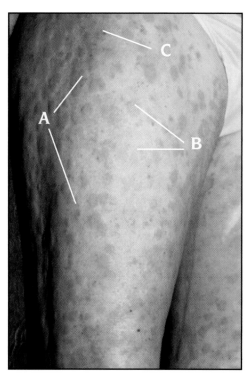

Figure 6: Urticarial Vasculitis involving the thighs. (A) wheals are raised; (B) associated bruise-like appearance as hives resolve; (C) small blue-purplish hemorrhages.

APPENDIX 1

CONDITIONS THAT MASQUERADE AS HIVES (URTICARIA) AND/OR SWELLING (ANGIOEDEMA)

A diagnosis of hives (urticaria) requires not only recognizing its major clinical characteristics (chapter 2), but also excluding skin conditions sometimes mistaken for hives. The following are some of these skin conditions.

GENERALIZED ITCHING: Some patients believe they have hives because their skin is itchy. If they have been scratching their skin for a long time, the skin appears thickened and leathery. More frequently, the itchy skin is not associated with a rash. The important point is that other features of hives described in **chapter 2** must accompany itching in order to make a diagnosis of hives.

It is worth noting that chronic itching is usually a benign condition associated with dry skin or anxiety. However, it can be associated with illnesses, such as systemic drug reactions, low thyroid condition, liver disease, kidney disorders, diabetes, polycythemia vera, scabies, and certain cancers, such as lymphomas. A full medical evaluation may be required for persistent itching.

ECZEMA: Occasionally, some patients confuse this condition with hives. Classic allergic eczema is a chronic, itchy, rash involving the flexing skin locations of elbow and knee joints, cheeks, hands, tops of large toes, and other regions of the body. Eczema is associated with inflamed, swollen and sometimes thickened skin that may persist at the same location for weeks or longer. There are many causes of eczema, including allergic factors (animal exposure; food sensitivity), and chemicals that cause eczema by direct skin contact.

Except for the observation that hives and eczema are associated with itching, there is no other similarity between these conditions, especially since hives do not persist at the same location for more than 24 to 36 hours.

INSECT BITES: Insect bites from spiders or other small insects may produce a rash that is occasionally confused with hives. The confusion is natural since insect bites may contain histamine that will produce small, pimple-sized welts with reddened borders. Usually insect bites cause inflammatory skin reactions that will remain for several days at the same location. In contrast, hives do not remain at the same location for more than 24 to 36 hours. Insect bites also tend to cluster, as insects may bite or sting several times at the same location.

BLISTERS: A blister is a sac filled with clear fluid that may be caused by abrasions or infections. The overlying skin is thin and can easily be broken, allowing clear fluid to ooze out. A hive is covered by thicker skin, which cannot easily be broken. Blisters caused by inflammatory responses to infections or other serious skin conditions are referred to as **bullous-vesicular** lesions. These lesions require immediate attention from a dermatologist.

ACNE: One of the more common rashes occasionally confused with hives is acne. Acne can have multiple appearances, but in general, the rash is typically raised, red, and sometimes pus-like inflamed pimples. The pus-like inflamed appearance is occasionally confused with hives. The important difference is acne remains unchanged for more than 24 to 36 hours at the same location and is typically not itchy.

The next two entities may be difficult for healthcare professionals to differentiate from hives. The most important distinguishing feature of these conditions is both rashes remain essentially unchanged in the same location after 24 or 36 hours.

ERYTHEMA MULTIFORME (E.M): This term refers to a generally benign condition that on rare conditions can become systemic and life-threatening. **Erythema** refers to redness and **multiforme** means different shapes and sizes. Literally, it describes a red rash of many sizes and shapes. This condition has several features that should enable it to be separated from true hives.

The rash is raised, red, usually has no wheals, and generally is not itchy. The rash may have a bull's-eye target appearance, (**figure 5 in the color section of this book**). It initially involves the more peripheral parts of the body such as the hands, feet, and face. Gradually, over days or longer, the rash may progress to more central regions, such as the chest and abdomen. It is occasionally preceded by a history of body and joint aches, fever, and fatigue, all of which are suggestive of an underlying infectious illness. Some cases of E.M. are actually caused by viral infections, such as Herpes Simplex virus, which also causes cold sores. Occasional cases are caused by drug reactions (to sulfa and penicillin) and more rarely, by underlying malignancies that may be associated with this condition.

The major differences from classic hives are:

- E.M. persists and remains essentially unchanged at the same location for more than 24 or 36 hours, compared to true hives, which fade away within that time interval.

- E.M. is frequently preceded by fever, joint pains and fatigue.

- E.M. first affects peripheral parts of the body, such as the face, hands and feet.

At times, there is an overlap between these conditions, as E.M. may occasionally have a wheal-like appearance, necessitating assistance from a healthcare professional with allergy or dermatology expertise. On rare occasions, E.M. may become a systemic life-threatening condition requiring immediate medical attention, especially if patients develop swelling, sores or ulcers inside the mouth.

URTICARIAL VASCULITIS (U.V.): FIGURE 6 IN THE COLOR SECTION OF THIS BOOK. This is one of the most important rashes that needs to be differentiated from true hives. This condition includes wheals but differs from hives, as the rash remains unchanged for more than 24 or 36 hours in the same location. It may be associated with serious underlying diseases.

The rash of U.V. differs from true hives because it:

- is less itchy and more painful than hives.

- is more prominent on the legs, especially the lower legs.

- may be associated with small, blue-purple hemorrhages and bruises that become noticeable as the rash resolves over weeks or longer.

- is occasionally associated with multi-systemic symptoms, such as joint pains, fever, inflammation of the eye (uveitis), respiratory symptoms of chronic obstructive lung disease (COPD), kidney involvement, nervous system symptoms, abdominal pain, etc.

- It remains unchanged for more than 24 or 36 hours at the same location.

- The wheals of U.V. feel hard to the touch compared to the softness of true hives (urticaria).

U.V. can be associated with serious systemic underlying disorders, such as lupus erythematosus, rheumatoid arthritis, hepatitis, serum sickness, cryoglobulinemia and malignancies. The laboratory evaluation for U.V. should include CBC, ESR, chemistries, total complement (CH_{50} with classic complement components C_3, C_4, C_1), cryoglobulin, C_{1q} autoantibody, serum protein electrophoresis, ANA panel and skin biopsy. The diagnosis can be made on the basis of a skin biopsy and evidence of classic component complement utilization, although there are forms of U.V with normal complement blood levels.

A diagnosis of swelling (angioedema) requires recognizing not only its major characteristics (chapter 2), but also excluding conditions that may masquerade as angioedema. The following conditions may be mistaken for angioedema.

FLUID OVERLOAD refers to clinical conditions in which patients become swollen due to excess fluid and/or salt intake. This is more commonly observed in a hospital environment when patients inadvertently receive excess intravenous fluids, but occasionally occurs when individuals ingest unusually large volumes of fluids after vigorous activities. "**Fluid overload swelling**" is generally symmetrical and can be associated with pain, especially if rings cannot be removed. Pushing down with a fingertip will leave an indentation that may last for many seconds. This differs from angioedema, in which a similar maneuver leaves a very transient indentation. Also, angioedema is often asymmetrical, while fluid load-swelling is generally symmetrical.

TRAUMA can cause swelling in deep anatomical compartments under the skin. Sometimes "**trauma-induced swelling**" is not obvious by history and examination. For example, I evaluated a patient who was referred for swelling that occurred during a root canal procedure. The dentist irrigated the root canal with a medicinal agent and within minutes her lower right jaw swelled. She developed asymmetrical deep tissue swelling that was painful, and met almost all the criteria to make a diagnosis of angioedema. Over a period of ten hours, progressive black and blue discoloration developed around her swollen jaw. It became apparent the swelling was caused by a ruptured blood vessel that caused blood to leak into deep anatomical compartments in the lower jaw. The associated black and blue discoloration reflected the presence of blood beneath the skin. Swelling with bruises is diagnostic of trauma-induced swelling and differentiates it from angioedema.

VENOUS DISORDERS: Obstruction of blood flow from a blood clot or inflammation of a vein may cause thrombophlebitis, more commonly referred to as phlebitis. **"Phlebitis swelling"** may last days or longer, thus distinguishing it from angioedema, which resolves within less than 72 hours. The swelling is often painful. Pushing down on the swelling of phlebitis will leave an indentation that can remain for many seconds. This differs from angioedema, in which a similar maneuver leaves a very transient indentation.

Elderly people can develop swelling of the legs and feet due to varicose veins. **"Varicose vein swelling"** will remain indefinitely, distinguishing it from angioedema, which improves within 72 hours. Pushing down on the swelling due to varicose veins will leave an indentation that can remain for many seconds.

Some individuals may notice symmetrical swelling of their hands, fingers or feet at the end of a walk or run or after sitting for prolonged periods, such as during travel. This swelling is caused by pooling of venous blood in dependent parts of the body, and usually disappears an hour or two after termination of the activity that caused the swelling. The symmetrical swelling and rapid improvement of **"venous swelling"** within hours distinguishes it from angioedema.

Veins can be compressed by tumors, fractured bones, and hemorrhages, all of which can lead to chronic deep swelling of tissues. Compression of large veins in the chest can cause chronic swelling of the face and neck. I evaluated a fifty-year old female who was referred with a three-month history of persistent swelling of her face and neck. She treated herself for a month with vitamins and herbs and then saw her healthcare professional who made the diagnosis of angioedema. She received several cortisone injections, namely triamcinolone, (Kenalog®) over a two-month period, but the symptoms persisted. She was subsequently referred for a second opinion and it was apparent that the **"vein compression swelling"** was very different from angioedema because it was symmetrical and persistent. In addition, her vein compression-swelling was not responsive to cortisone, while angioedema often improves with that treatment. A chest X-ray revealed the presence of a tumor that compressed large veins in her neck and chest. Unfortunately, the cancerous tumor was not operable, partly because of the delay in diagnosis, and she died shortly thereafter.

LOW THYROID ASSOCIATED CONDITIONS: Individuals with hypothyroidism may notice swelling around their eyes, face and lower legs, specifically over their anterior tibia.

In contrast to angioedema, "**low thyroid-induced swelling**" persists for months until the condition is treated with thyroid hormone medication. Patients with low thyroid may notice fatigue, weight gain, thinning hair and irregular menstrual cycles.

PAROTID GLAND OBSTRUCTION: Parotid gland ducts can be obstructed by mineral stones, tumors and inflammation induced by an infectious disease (mumps). When the duct is blocked for whatever cause, the parotid gland may swell, which will create an asymmetrical appearance of the face. On occasion, asymmetrical parotid swelling may be confused with angioedema. "**Parotid duct obstruction swelling**" will frequently last many days or weeks compared to the shorter duration of angioedema.

CHRONIC SKIN INFLAMMATION: Almost all chronic, itchy skin conditions are associated with an inflammatory component that may include some degree of swelling. Examples include allergic types of eczema, chemical-induced eczema, and chronic skin infections caused by insect mites (scabies), bacteria (impetigo), and fungal organisms (ringworm). Unfortunately, the scope of this handbook does not permit a discussion of all inflammatory skin conditions. Compared to the one to three day swelling associated with angiodema, "**chronic skin inflammatory-induced swelling**" is almost always persistent and lasts until the skin condition is treated.

AUTOIMMUNE CONDITIONS: Autoimmune conditions refer to disease states in which individuals develop antibodies to their own cells and tissues. A number of autoimmune conditions can present with swelling of the skin. Lupus erythematosus is an autoimmune condition that can cause puffiness and redness of skin areas exposed to sunlight. Dermatomyositis, a condition involving skin and skeletal muscles, is associated with puffiness and swelling of the face and hands. "**Autoimmune-induced swelling**" is associated with persistent puffiness and swelling and can be differentiated from angioedema on that basis.

LYMPHATIC OBSTRUCTION: Any condition that causes obstruction and/or interruption of lymphatic ducts will cause leakage of lymph fluid beneath the surface of the skin resulting in "**lymphedema swelling**". Causes include lymph node tumors (lymphomas, such as Hodgkin's disease), post-operative lymphedema following radical breast surgery ,and parasitic infections that are prevalent in third world countries. In general, lymphedema will persist for weeks or longer, differentiating it from angioedema.

MELKERSSON-ROSENTHAL SYNDROME is a rare condition that mimics angioedema, as it is associated with swelling of the lip. Persistent chronic swelling for weeks or longer separates it from classic angioedema. Other symptoms include facial palsy and furrowed tongue. Biopsy of the involved lip swelling reveals granulomatous inflammation.

APPENDIX 2

COMPLETING
DIARIES

Purpose: The evaluation of hives and/or swelling is usually based on the history and physical examination. The purpose of this exercise is to make detailed daily observations of skin symptoms to detect unrecognized triggers of hives and/or swelling.

Explanation: There are many factors that can influence and cause hives and/or swelling. One way to uncover possible triggers is to keep a detailed diary. At the same time each day, patients rate the severity of their hives and/or swelling using the severity rating scale listed at the bottom of the diary page. Record should include:

- The time when there is an increase in the severity rating of hives and/or swelling.
- If there is an increase in severity rating.
- Foods eaten, medications taken, activities and other symptoms occurring during the 2 hour interval prior to increase in severity.

Review the diary to determine whether there are external triggers that may be causing or exacerbating skin symptoms. The review should note whether the severity of symptoms increases in relation to any of the following factors:

- Taking a medication, such as an NSAID.
- Following the ingestion of a food.
- During exercise, physical exertion or other activities.
- Indoors or outdoors.
- Nighttime or daytime.
- Exposure to cold or hot environments.

Each trigger can be a clue to a potential cause, which can be researched using the index in this text.

I recommend filling out daily diaries for a minimum of one week. The backside of each diary page can be used to detail information, such as food ingredients.

INSTRUCTIONS: Record Hive and Swelling ratings upon awakening. (See Ratings below.) If there is an increase in rating during day or night, record time with new rating, all foods eaten, medications taken, and activities FOR THE TWO (2) HOURS PRIOR TO THE INCREASE IN SYMPTOMS.

NAME: _____   DATE: _____

Time	Hive Rating (+) Swelling Rating (++)	Medications (*)	Foods Eaten (#)	Activities (^)	Other Physical Issues (~)

+ **Hive rating is the number of hives. Record rating from previous day and record only increase in rating score.**
　　Scale: **0**=none; **1**=1-5 hives; **2**=6-10 hives; **3**=11-20 hives; **4**=more than 20 hives

++ **Swelling rating is the number of swellings. Record rating from previous day and record only increase in rating score.**
　　Scale: **0**=none; **1**=1 swelling; **2**=2 swellings; **3**=3 swellings; **4**=4 or more swellings.

* **Medications include all prescriptions, over-the-counter medications, alternative medications etc. by any method of administration.**

Please list details of foods with ingredients on the back of this chart.

~ **List any unusual symptoms, like hoarseness, headache, joint pains, abdominal pains, etc.**

^ **Activities: Include exercise (indoors or outdoors); sexual activity; other such as prolonged sitting, standing, using tools, etc.**

INSTRUCTIONS: Record Hive and Swelling ratings upon awakening. (See Ratings below.) If there is an increase in rating during day or night, record time with new rating, all foods eaten, medications taken, and activities FOR THE TWO (2) HOURS PRIOR TO THE INCREASE IN SYMPTOMS.

NAME: _____   DATE: _____

Time	Hive Rating (+) Swelling Rating (++)	Medications (*)	Foods Eaten (#)	Activities (^)	Other Physical Issues (~)

+ Hive rating is the number of hives. Record rating from previous day and record only increase in rating score.
   Scale: **0**=none; **1**=1-5 hives; **2**=6-10 hives; **3**=11-20 hives; **4**=more than 20 hives

++ Swelling rating is the number of swellings. Record rating from previous day and record only increase in rating score.
   Scale: **0**=none; **1**=1 swelling; **2**=2 swellings; **3**=3 swellings; **4**=4 or more swellings.

* Medications include all prescriptions, over-the-counter medications, alternative medications etc. by any method of administration.

 # Please list details of foods with ingredients on the back of this chart.

~ List any unusual symptoms, like hoarseness, headache, joint pains, abdominal pains, etc.

^ Activities: Include exercise (indoors or outdoors); sexual activity; other such as prolonged sitting, standing, using tools, etc.

INSTRUCTIONS: Record Hive and Swelling ratings upon awakening. (See Ratings below.) If there is an increase in rating during day or night, record time with new rating, all foods eaten, medications taken, and activities FOR THE TWO (2) HOURS PRIOR TO THE INCREASE IN SYMPTOMS.

NAME: _____   DATE: _____

Time	Hive Rating (+) Swelling Rating (++)	Medications (*)	Foods Eaten (#)	Activities (^)	Other Physical Issues (~)

+   Hive rating is the number of hives. Record rating from previous day and record only increase in rating score.
    Scale: **0**=none; **1**=1-5 hives; **2**=6-10 hives; **3**=11-20 hives; **4**=more than 20 hives

++   Swelling rating is the number of swellings. **Record rating from previous day and record only increase in rating score.**
    Scale: **0**=none; **1**=1 swelling: **2**=2 swellings; **3**=3 swellings; **4**=4 or more swellings.

*   **Medications include all prescriptions, over-the-counter medications, alternative medications etc. by any method of administration.**

Please list details of foods with ingredients on the back of this chart.

~   List any unusual symptoms, like hoarseness, headache, joint pains, abdominal pains, etc.

^   **Activities: Include exercise (indoors or outdoors); sexual activity; other such as prolonged sitting, standing, using tools, etc.**

INSTRUCTIONS: Record Hive and Swelling ratings upon awakening. (See Ratings below.) If there is an increase in rating during day or night, record time with new rating, all foods eaten, medications taken, and activities FOR THE TWO (2) HOURS PRIOR TO THE INCREASE.IN SYMPTOMS.

NAME: _____   DATE: _____

Time	Hive Rating (+) Swelling Rating (++)	Medications (*)	Foods Eaten (#)	Activities (^)	Other Physical Issues (~)

+   **Hive rating is the number of hives. Record rating from previous day and record only increase in rating score.**

     Scale: **0**=none; **1**=1-5 hives; **2**=6-10 hives; **3**=11-20 hives; **4**=more than 20 hives

++   **Swelling rating is the number of swellings. Record rating from previous day and record only increase in rating score.**

     Scale: **0**=none; **1**=1 swelling; **2**=2 swellings; **3**=3 swellings; **4**=4 or more swellings.

*   **Medications include all prescriptions, over-the-counter medications, alternative medications etc. by any method of administration.**

Please list details of foods with ingredients on the back of this chart.

~   List any unusual symptoms, like hoarseness, headache, joint pains, abdominal pains, etc.

^   Activities: Include exercise (indoors or outdoors); sexual activity; other such as prolonged sitting, standing, using tools, etc.

INSTRUCTIONS: Record Hive and Swelling ratings upon awakening. (See Ratings below.) If there is an increase in rating during day or night, record time with new rating, all foods eaten, medications taken, and activities FOR THE TWO (2) HOURS PRIOR TO THE INCREASE.IN SYMPTOMS.

NAME: _____   DATE: _____

Time	Hive Rating (+) Swelling Rating (++)	Medications (*)	Foods Eaten (#)	Activities (^)	Other Physical Issues (~)

+ **Hive rating is the number of hives. Record rating from previous day and record only increase in rating score.**
Scale: **0**=none; **1**=1-5 hives; **2**=6-10 hives; **3**=11-20 hives; **4**=more than 20 hives

++ **Swelling rating is the number of swellings. Record rating from previous day and record only increase in rating score.**
Scale: **0**=none; **1**=1 swelling; **2**=2 swellings; **3**=3 swellings; **4**=4 or more swellings.

* **Medications include all prescriptions, over-the-counter medications, alternative medications etc. by any method of administration.**

Please list details of foods with ingredients on the back of this chart.

~ **List any unusual symptoms, like hoarseness, headache, joint pains, abdominal pains, etc.**

^ **Activities: Include exercise (indoors or outdoors); sexual activity; other such as prolonged sitting, standing, using tools, etc.**

INSTRUCTIONS: Record Hive and Swelling ratings upon awakening. (See Ratings below.) If there is an increase in rating during day or night, record time with new rating, all foods eaten, medications taken, and activities FOR THE TWO (2) HOURS PRIOR TO THE INCREASE IN SYMPTOMS.

NAME: _____   DATE: _____

Time	Hive Rating (+) Swelling Rating (++)	Medications (*)	Foods Eaten (#)	Activities (^)	Other Physical Issues (~)

+   Hive rating is the number of hives. Record rating from previous day and record only increase in rating score.
   Scale: 0=none; 1=1-5 hives; 2=6-10 hives; 3=11-20 hives; 4=more than 20 hives

++ Swelling rating is the number of swellings. Record rating from previous day and record only increase in rating score.
   Scale: 0=none; 1=1 swelling; 2=2 swellings; 3=3 swellings; 4=4 or more swellings.

*   Medications include all prescriptions, over-the-counter medications, alternative medications etc. by any method of administration.

 #   Please list details of foods with ingredients on the back of this chart.

~   List any unusual symptoms, like hoarseness, headache, joint pains, abdominal pains, etc.

APPENDIX 3

RECORD OF
EVALUATION AND TREATMENT

This appendix provides a template for recording the evaluation and treatment of H/S. It is particularly useful for following the care of patients with chronic H/S.

SUMMARY OF EVALUATION

■ **Documentation of urticaria** by physical examination (PE) or by photographs (PH). Yes_____ No _____

- If Yes, Date _____ Documentation by PE or PH _____
- Location of urticaria

■ **Documentation of angioedema** by physical examination (PE) or by photographs (PH). Yes_____ No_____

- If Yes, Date _____ Documentation by PE or PH_____
- Location of angioedema

■ **Documentation of urticaria disappearing within 24 to 36 hours.**

- Yes_____ No _____
- If Yes, was it documented by patient or by HCP?

    HCP_____ Patient _____

- **Documentation of angioedema disappearing within 72 hours.**

  - Yes_____ No _____
  - If Yes, was it documented by patient or by HCP ?

        HCP_____ Patient _____

- **Test for dermographism** using 0-4 scale (0 is negative and 4 is maximum).

  Result_____ Date _____

- **Test for other physical sensitivities**, if appropriate. Record (positive or negative):

  - **Cold stimulation test (#32)** Result _____ Date _____
  - **Deep pressure test(#30)** Result _____ Date _____
  - **Solar test (#31)** Result _____ Date _____
  - **Heat (#34)** Result_____ Date _____
  - **Exercise test (#33)**

        Exercise challenge Result_____ Date _____
        Intradermal Mecholyl® Result_____ Date _____
    Water (aquagenic) test (#35) Result _____ Date _____
    Misc. test Type _____ Result _____Date _____
    Misc. test Type _____ Result _____Date _____

- **Intradermal skin test** for circulating autoantibodies to IgE and/or IgE receptors **(# 84)**. Result _____ Date _____

- **General blood tests** such as chemistry screen, CBC, ESR etc:
  Date and Results

  _____

  _____

  _____

  _____

  _____

  _____

- **Repeat general blood tests:**
  Date and Results

  _____

  _____

  _____

  _____

- **Specific tests**, if appropriate

  - For **hereditary angioedema(#39)** Type of test_____ ;
    Result _____ Date _____
  - For **acquired angioedema (#26E)** Type of test_____
    Result _____ Date _____
  - For **autoimmune thyroiditis (#54,#55)** Type of test_____
    Result _____ Date _____
  - **Skin and/or IgE specific RAST tests**:
    For **foods(#52)** Type of test_____ Date _____
    List foods that are positive

    _____

    _____

    If positive, was a challenge performed? Yes___ No ____ Date _____
    Details of type of challenge _____

    For **medications (#50)** Type of test_____ Date _____
    List medications that are positive

    _____

    _____

    If positive, was a challenge performed? Yes___ No ____ Date _____
    Details of type of challenge _____

    For **insect venom(#51)** Type of test_____ Date _____
    List insect venom that was positive

    _____

    _____

For **latex (#42)** Type of test_____ Result_____Date _____

For **miscellaneous antigens** List antigens, type of test and result
Date _____

_____

_____

• **Patch tests** List antigens tested and results

_____

_____

• **Skin biopsy** List type of stain, results Date _____

_____

_____

Miscellaneous blood and/or other tests (X-rays, etc.)

Test _____ Date _____

Result _____

Test _____ Date _____

Result _____

Test _____ Date _____

Result _____

Test _____ Date _____

Result _____

• **Record any abnormal physical examination (PE)** observations that may be
relevant to the urticaria/angioedema:

PE abnormality_____ Date _____

PE abnormality_____ Date _____

PE abnormality_____ Date _____

PE abnormality_____ Date _____

TREATMENT RECORD

DATE	RX	DOSE	HISTAMINE SKIN TEST[+] (IF ON ANTI-HISTAMINE)	RX EFFECTIVENESS *
____	_____	_____	_____	_____
____	_____	_____	_____	_____
____	_____	_____	_____	_____
____	_____	_____	_____	_____
____	_____	_____	_____	_____
____	_____	_____	_____	_____
____	_____	_____	_____	_____
____	_____	_____	_____	_____
____	_____	_____	_____	_____
____	_____	_____	_____	_____
____	_____	_____	_____	_____
____	_____	_____	_____	_____
____	_____	_____	_____	_____
____	_____	_____	_____	_____
____	_____	_____	_____	_____
____	_____	_____	_____	_____
____	_____	_____	_____	_____
____	_____	_____	_____	_____
____	_____	_____	_____	_____
____	_____	_____	_____	_____
____	_____	_____	_____	_____
____	_____	_____	_____	_____

[+] A dosage adjustment or change of antihistamine may be advised if histamine test is very positive.

* Grade according to scoring system located on bottom of diary sheet (Appendix 2).

TREATMENT RECORD

DATE	RX	DOSE	HISTAMINE SKIN TEST[+] (IF ON ANTI-HISTAMINE)	RX EFFECTIVENESS *
___	_____	_____	_____	_____
___	_____	_____	_____	_____
___	_____	_____	_____	_____
___	_____	_____	_____	_____
___	_____	_____	_____	_____
___	_____	_____	_____	_____
___	_____	_____	_____	_____
___	_____	_____	_____	_____
___	_____	_____	_____	_____
___	_____	_____	_____	_____
___	_____	_____	_____	_____
___	_____	_____	_____	_____
___	_____	_____	_____	_____
___	_____	_____	_____	_____
___	_____	_____	_____	_____
___	_____	_____	_____	_____
___	_____	_____	_____	_____
___	_____	_____	_____	_____
___	_____	_____	_____	_____
___	_____	_____	_____	_____
___	_____	_____	_____	_____
___	_____	_____	_____	_____

[+] A dosage adjustment or change of antihistamine may be advised if histamine test is very positive.

* Grade according to scoring system located on bottom of diary sheet (Appendix 2).

GLOSSARY

Allergen: a foreign protein that can induce allergic IgE antibody responses.

Alpha tryptase: an enzyme released from mast cells which may be elevated in systemic mastocytosis.

Anaphylatoxins: by-products (C_{5a}, C_{5b}) of the complement system that can release chemical mediators from mast cells. The end result is the induction of hives and/or swelling.

Anaphylaxis: a severe systemic, allergic IgE-mediated reaction characterized by hives, swelling, difficulty breathing and possibly, shock and death.

ANA profile: an anti-nuclear antibody test for autoimmune diseases.

Angioedema: the medical term for swelling associated with immune mechanisms, non-immune mechanisms and other causes.

Antibodies: protein molecules produced by the immune system in response to antigens and allergens.

Antigen: molecules that induce an immune response, such as antibody production.

Anti-leukotrienes: medications that interfere in the biologic activity of a mediator called leukotrienes, either by reducing the production of leukotrienes or by blocking the action of leukotrienes.

Arthralgia: joint pains.

Autoantibodies: antibodies that are formed against normal cell components and can cause the development of autoimmune diseases. An example is lupus erythematosus in which antibodies are formed against DNA (chromosomes) in cells.

Autoimmune (Autoimmunity): Disorders caused by abnormal immune reactions to one's tissues or organs. Lupus erythematosus is an example in which antibodies to DNA (chromosomes) cause a multitude of symptoms involving the blood, central nervous system, heart, kidneys and other organ systems.

185

Autosomal co-dominant: a disease pattern of inheritance in which 50% of multi-generational family members are affected. The pattern affects females and males equally.

Beta tryptase: an enzyme that can be released from mast cells during anaphylactic reactions. The elevation of beta tryptase can document anaphylactic reactions.

Bone scan: a radiological technique which combines radioisotope injection with bone X-rays.

Bradykinin: a by-product of the blood clotting system that has mediator properties and may cause swelling and/or hives.

Bronchiectasis: a chronic lung disease caused by repeated infections.

BUN: **b**lood **u**rea **n**itrogen measurement, a test of kidney function. If elevated, it may represent decreased kidney function, but may also be elevated for other reasons, such as dehydration and bleeding in the intestinal tract.

C_1 esterase inhibitor: a protein that controls the complement pathway. If it is quantitatively low or functionally abnormal it can be responsible for hereditary types of angioedema.

C_{1q}: a component of complement which if decreased, may indicate a diagnosis of acquired angioedema.

C_{1q} assay: see solid C_{1q} assay.

C_4: a component of complement which if decreased, may indicate a diagnosis of hereditary or acquired angioedema.

CBC: **c**omplete **b**lood **c**ount that includes a white blood cell count, cell differential, platelet count, and other measurements.

Celiac disease: an intestinal disease characterized by decreased absorption of nutrients caused by sensitivity to gluten in wheat and other grains.

Cell mediated immunity: immune responses associated with types of white blood cells called lymphocytes.

CH_{50}: 50% of total complement level.

Chemokines: chemical messengers released by various cells that attract other cells to the site of an inflammatory reaction. Chemokines are released as part of the chronic inflammation that results in hives.

Chemistry screen: chemistry tests that measure function of various organ systems.

COPD: abbreviation for **c**hronic **o**bstructive **p**ulmonary (lung) **d**isease characterized by reduced lung function. Generally, the airflow is obstructed due to chronic inflammation caused by toxins, immune reactions, and infections.

Cold agglutinin: a test that indirectly detects mycoplasma infection.

Common variable immunodeficiency (CVID): A deficiency of the immune system characterized by reduced immunoglobulin levels. Patients may experience recurring infections involving the sinuses, ears, lungs, and the intestinal tract.

Complement: a group of serum proteins involved in the control of inflammation and the activation of white blood cells that engulf and destroy infectious agents. Complement activation can be detected by measuring total complement (CH_{50}).

Creatinine clearance: a blood and urine test that measures kidney function.

Cryoglobulin: an abnormal protein in the blood that may precipitate out of blood under cold conditions.

C Urea breath test: detects *Helicobacter pylori* infection involving the stomach.

Cystoscopy: endoscopy of the bladder.

Dysproteinemia: an abnormal elevation of antibody proteins sometimes associated with cancers of the blood or lymphatic systems.

Electromyography: muscle testing using electrical stimulation.

Endoscopy: a procedure in which a fiberoptic tube is inserted into an anatomical opening to view internal tissue and sometimes obtain a tissue specimen for biopsy.

Eosinophil count: a type of white blood cell that can be elevated in IgE allergic mechanisms. Eosinophil counts may also be elevated in non-IgE-mediated responses.

Erythema or erythematous: redness of the skin or skin lesion.

ESR: erythrocyte **s**edimentation **r**ate. A non-specific test for inflammation caused by many conditions, such as infections and autoimmune diseases.

Furunculosis: a skin condition caused by bacterial infections.

Gammopathy: an abnormal elevation of antibody protein sometimes associated with cancer of the bone marrow.

Giemsa stain: a dye used to stain for mast cells in skin biopsies. An increased number of mast cells suggests the diagnosis of urticaria pigmentosa or mastocytosis.

Gingivitis: inflammation of the gums.

Glomerulonephritis: an inflammatory condition of the kidneys that affects the filtering units that produce urine.

Granulomatous: a type of tissue inflammation that is considered chronic.

H$_1$ receptor: histamine receptors in the skin that bind histamine and cause itching and swelling.

H$_2$ receptor: histamine receptors in the stomach and skin. The histamine effect on H$_2$ receptors in the stomach is acid production. H$_2$ receptor effects in the skin are similar to those of H$_1$ receptors.

H & E: a specific stain (hematoxylin and eosin), which is used for staining tissue specimens for microscopic examination.

Helicobacter pylori: a bacterium that causes stomach ulcers. It has been implicated as a cause of chronic hives.

Herpes Simplex Virus: a virus that can cause cold sores and a condition called erythema multiforme that may masquerade as hives.

Herpes zoster: a viral infectious agent that causes shingles.

Hepatitis A, B, C screen: blood tests to detect infections with these three types of hepatitis virus.

HLA typing: The identification of specific markers (antigens) on the surface of white blood cells. A characteristic pattern of markers is observed for rheumatoid arthritis and other diseases that have hereditary influences, such as familial dermographism.

Humoral immune system: the branch of immune system that produces antibodies (see immunoglobulin).

Idiopathic: of unknown cause.

IgE: a class of immunoglobulin that includes allergic antibodies in the blood.

Immunofluorescent stains: a microscopy technique that provides information regarding the presence of immune proteins in tissue specimens. Specific patterns may verify the diagnosis of conditions, such as lupus erythematosus.

Immunologist: a specialist of the immune system.

Immunoglobulin (Ig): antibody proteins that are produced by the immune system. There are five classes of immunoglobulin and each one has separate functions. IgE represents allergic antibodies; IgG represents the largest quantity of antibodies that control infections; IgM represents a class composed of larger molecules of immunoglobulin that are produced in the early response against infectious agents; and IgA is a class that is produced in saliva, tears and other secretions.

Interstitial cystitis: an inflammatory disorder of the bladder of unknown cause that is associated with frequent and painful urination.

KOH scraping: a procedure in which skin is scraped onto a slide and KOH (potassium hydroxide) is added to visualize the presence of fungal organisms under a microscope.

Leukotrienes: chemical mediators that can cause hives and/or swelling.

Mast cells: specialized cells located in the skin and internal organs which contain chemicals (histamine) that can cause hives and/or swelling.

Mediators: chemicals that are manufactured and stored in mast cells. A hive or wheal develops when mediators cause leakage of plasma (water, electrolytes such as sodium and potassium, and protein) through the walls of small blood vessels into the skin.

Mono test: a blood test to detect infectious mononucleosis.

Mycoplasma: an infectious agent that affects the respiratory tract.

Nephrologist: a medical specialist of the kidney system.

Neurologist: a medical specialist of the nerve and muscle systems.

Parathyroid hormone test: a blood assay that measures the level of a hormone produced by a gland located in the neck. This hormone is involved in controlling calcium and phosphorus metabolism.

Papular urticaria: Pimple-shaped hives.

Patch tests: the application of substances on the surface of the skin to test for sensitivity. In most circumstances, this test remains in place for 48-72 hours to detect delayed skin contact reactions. However, in contact urticaria, a similar test can be done and then removed 15-30 minutes after application. A test that induces wheal production within 30 minutes of application is suggestive of an IgE allergic mechanism.

Periocular: around the eye.

Perioxidase and Thyroglobulin anti-thyroid antibodies: antibodies associated with autoimmune thyroiditis (inflammation of the thyroid, called Hashimoto's disease).

Platelet activating factor: a mediator that can cause hives and/or swelling.

Polycythemia vera: a blood disease associated with unexplained elevation of red blood cells.

Polymyositis: an inflammatory disorder of muscles that causes muscle pain and weakness.

Progesterone: a female hormone produced by the ovaries.

Prostaglandins: a group of chemicals manufactured in various cells. A few types of prostaglandins can cause hives and/or swelling.

Protoscopy and colonoscopy: endoscopy tests of the rectum and colon.

Pruritis or pruritic: itchiness, or itchy.

PSA: **p**rostate **s**pecific **a**ntigen blood test that may detect prostate cancer.

Pulmonary function: lung tests that measure breathing function.

Raji equivalent C_{3D} assay: a test that may detect the presence of circulating immune complexes (mixtures of antigen, antibody and complement) involved in causing illnesses, such as serum sickness and autoimmune diseases.

RAST: a blood test for IgE (allergic antibody) to a specific allergen. The acronym stands for radioallergosorbent test.

Rheumatoid factor: a blood test that suggests the presence of autoantibodies characteristic of rheumatoid arthritis.

Serum protein immunoelectrophoresis: a blood test that separates serum proteins by the application of an electrical charge. It may detect abnormal elevations of serum antibody proteins associated with certain types of cancers.

Serum immunofixation: a refinement of serum protein electrophoresis that can identify individual classes of antibodies.

Solid C_{1q} assay: a test that may detect the presence of circulating immune complexes (mixtures of antigen, antibody and complement) involved in causing illnesses, such as serum sickness and autoimmune diseases.

Stool for ova and parasites: a microscopic test on fecal specimens for parasites or parasite eggs.

Sjogren antibody test: measures antibodies associated with Sjogren's syndrome, which is an autoimmune disorder.

Streptozyme test: detects streptococcal infections.

Tear volume: measures tear volume that is reduced in Sjogren's syndrome. Reduced tear volume is responsible for dry eyes that are associated with this syndrome.

Thyroid function tests: a group of blood tests that measure thyroid function and may include free thyroid hormone (T_4), Thyroid Stimulating Hormone (TSH) and thyroid autoantibodies (antibodies that cause inflammation of the thyroid).

Toluidine blue: a dye used to stain for mast cells in skin biopsies. An increased number of mast cells suggests the diagnosis of urticaria pigmentosa or mastocytosis.

Urologist: a medical specialist of the urinary tract system.

Urticaria: the medical term for hives.

Uveitis: inflammation of the uvea located in the eye.

REFERENCES

General background and mechanisms

1. Black AK. Unusual urticarias. J Dermatol 200;28(11):632-4.
2. Charlesworth EN. Differential diagnosis of angioedema. Allergy Asthma Proc 2002;23:337-339.
3. Charlesworth EN. Chronic urticaria: background, evaluation and treatment. Curr Allergy Asthma Rep 200;1(4):342-347.
4. Charlesworth EN. Urticaria. In: Charlesworth EN, ed. Immunology and Allergy Clinics of North America 1995;15:641-801.
5. Grattan CE, Sabroe RA, Greaves MW. Chronic urticaria. J Am Acad Dermatol 2002;46(5):645-57.
6. Greaves MW. Pathophysiology of chronic urticaria. Int Arch Allergy Immunol 2002;127(1):3-9.
7. Greaves MW. Current concepts: chronic urticaria. N Eng J Med 1995; 332:1767-71.
8. Greaves MW, O'Donnell BF. Not all chronic urticaria is idiopathic. Exp Dermatol 1998;7:11-13.
9. Gross AS, LaTour DL, King LE. Chronic urticaria: a model questionnaire for patient screening. Cutis 1990;46:421-444.
10. Henz BM, Zuberbier T, Grabbe J, et al., eds., Urticaria. Berlin Heidelberg-New York: Springer-Verlag, 1998.
11. Kaplan AP. Chronic urticaria and angioedema. N Eng J Med 2002;346(3):175-179.
12. Kaplan AP, Kusuman J, Silverberg M. Pathways for bradykinin formation and inflammatory disease. J Allergy Clin Immunol 2002;109:195-207.
13. Kaplan AP. Urticaria and angioedema. In: Middleton E, Reed CE, Ellis EF, et al., eds., Allergy, Principles and Practice (5th ed)., 1104-1122, 1998.
14. Kikuchi Y, Kaplan AP. A role for C5a in augmenting IgG-dependent histamine release from basophils in chronic urticaria. J Allergy Clin Immunol 2002;109:114-118.
15. Monte T. Hives. The Complete Guide to Natural Healing. Berkley publishing company, 1997.
16. Powell J, Powell S. Mechanisms underlying urticaria. Hosp Med 2000;61:470-474.
17. Tharp M. Chronic urticaria: pathophysiology and treatment approaches. J Allergy Clin Immunol 1996;98:S325-30.

18. Sabroe RA, Fiebiger E, Francis DM, et al. Classification of anti-FcERI and anti-IgE autoantibodies in chronic idiopathic urticaria and correlation with disease severity. J Allergy Clin Immunol 2002;110:491-499.

19. Van Dellen R, Maddox DE, Dutta EJ. Masqueraders of angioedema and urticaria. Ann Allergy Asthma Immunol 2002;88:10-14.

20. van der Valk PG, Moret G, Kiemeney LA. The natural history of chronic urticaria and angioedema in patients visiting a tertiary referral centre. Br J Dermatol 2002; 146(1):110-3.

21. Wanderer AA, Bernstein LB, Goodman DL, et al. The diagnosis and management of urticaria: a practice parameter. Ann Allergy Asthma Immunol 2000; 85(6):532-544.

22. Zuberbier T, Greaves MW, Juhlin L, et al. Definition, classification, and routine diagnosis of urticaria: a consensus report. J Inv Dermatol 2001;6:123-127.

(#9) Fever

1. Abraham D, Saltoun CA. Facial swelling and eosinophilia in a 44-year old woman. Ann Allergy Asthma Immunol 2002; 89:561-564.

2. Gleich GL, Schroeter AL, Marcoux JP, et al. Episodic angioedema associated with eosinophilia. N Eng J Med 1984;310(25):1621-1626.

3. Kohler PF. Clinical immune complex disease. Manifestations in systemic lupus erythematosus and hepatitis B virus infection. Medicine (Baltimore) 1973; 52(5):419-29.

4. Lipsker D, Spehner D, Drillien R, et al. Schnitzler's syndrome: heterogenous immunopathological findings involving IgM-skin interactions. Br J Dermatol 2000; 142:954-959.

(#10) Weight gain

1. Gleich GL, Schroeter AL, Marcoux JP, et al. Episodic angioedema associated with eosinophilia. N Eng J Med 1984;310(25):1621-1626.

2. Kandell AA, Zeid M, Helm T, et al. Evaluation of chronic urticaria in patients with Hashimoto's thyroiditis. J Clin Immunol 2001;21(5):335-447.

3. Leznoff A, Josse RG, Denburg J, et al. Association of chronic urticaria and angioedema with thyroid autoimmunity. Arch Dermatol 1983;119:636-640.

4. Rumbyrt JS, Katz JL, Schocket AL. Resolution of chronic urticaria in patients with thyroid autoimmunity. J Allergy Clin Immunol 1995;96:901-905.

(#12) Emotional symptoms

1. Haustein UF. Adrenergic urticaria and adrenergic pruritis. Acta Derm Venereol 1990;70(1):82-84.

2. Shelley WB, Shelley ED. Adrenergic urticaria: a new form of stress-induced hives. Lancet North Am Ed 1985;2:1031-1033.

3. Vithayasai P, Vithayasai V. Adrenergic urticaria: a first report from Thailand. J Med Assoc Thai 1989;72(8):478-480.

(#16,#17) Teeth are painful

1. Sonada T, Anan T, Ono K, et al. Chronic urticaria associated with dental infection. Br J Dermatol 2001;145(3):516-518.

(#18) Puffiness around the eyes

1. DeGroot AC. Patch testing: test concentrations and vehicles for 3700 chemicals (2nd ed). Amsterdam, NY: Elsevier, 1994.

(#19) Severe sore throat; difficulty swallowing; recurring hoarseness

1. Fremeaux-Bacchi V, Guinnepain MT, Cacoub P, et al. Prevalence of monoclonal gammopathy in patients presenting with acquired angioedema type 2. Am J Med 2002;113(3):249-51.

(#23A) Bone pain

1. Govindaraju S, Brochet P, Ringot AC, et al. Chronic urticaria-macroglobulinemia (Schnitzler's syndrome): developing to IgM myeloma. Apropos of a case. Rev Med Interne 1993;14(8):780-783.

(#24) Multiple bone fractures

1. Armstrong JL. Chronic idiopathic (?) urticaria: a satisfactory outcome. Ann Allergy Asthma Immunol 1999;83:95-98.
2. Dagher HN, Aboujaoude ZC, Jabbour SA: Chronic urticaria: an unusual initial manifestation of primary hyperparathyroidism. Endoc Pract 2002; 8:47-49.
3. Liechty RD, Firminger HI. Hyperparathyroidism and urticaria. JAMA 1983;250: 789-790.

(#26) Gastrointestinal

1. Dauden E, Jimenez-Alonso I, Garcia-Diez A. *Helicobacter pylori* and idiopathic chronic urticaria. Int J Dermatol 2000;39(6):446-52.
2. Hook-Nikanne J, Varjonen E, Harvima RJ et al. Is *Helicobacter pylori* infection associated with chronic urticaria? Acta Derm Venereol 2000;80(6):425-426.
3. Kohler PF. Clinical immune complex disease. Manifestations in systemic lupus erythematosus and hepatitis B virus infection. Medicine (Baltimore) 1973; 52(5):419-29.
4. Levine A, Dalal I, Bujanover Y. Celiac disease associated with a familial chronic urticaria and thyroid autoimmunity in a child. Pediatrics 1999;104(2):e25.
5. McKnight JT, Tietze PE. Dermatologic manifestations of giardiasis. J Am Board Fam Pract 1992;5(4):425-428.

6. Naimeh LG, Muller BA. Chronic urticaria in a 17-year-old patient with a past history of bowel disease. Ann Allergy Asthma Immunol 2001;86(5):511-516.

7. Ojetti V, Armuzzi A, DeLuca A, et al. *Helicobacter pylori* infection affects eosinophilic cationic protein in the gastric juice of patients with idiopathic chronic urticaria. Int Arch Allergy Immunol 2001;125(1):66-72.

8. Ortiz GG, Agustin MC, Martinez PE, et al. Chronic urticaria and *Helicobacter pylori*. Ann Allergy Asthma Immunol 2001;86:694-698.

9. Seth AK, Nair S, Singh J, et al. Hereditary angioedema with recurrent abdominal pain. Indian J Gastroenterol 2002; 21(2): 82-83.

10. Scala E, Giani M, Pirrotta L, et al. Urticaria and adult celiac disease. Allergy 1999; 54(9):1008-1009.

11. Scully LJ, Ryan AE. Urticaria and acute hepatitis A virus infection. Am J Gastroenterol 1993;88(2):277-278.

(#27) Urinary and reproductive systems (see also #76 below)

1. Jorgensen J, Weismann K: Urticaria in gonorrheal infection. Ugeskr Laeger 1987; 149(41):2795.

2. Lieberman J, Gephardt G, Calabrese LH: Urticaria, nephritis and pseudotumor cerebri. Cleve Clin J Med 1990; 57(2):197-210.

3. Moorthy AV, Pringle D. Urticaria vasculitis, hypocomplementemia, and immune-complex glomerulonephritis. Arch Pathol Lab Med 1982;106(2):68-70.

4. Sant GR, Theoharides TC, Letourneau R: Interstitial cystitis and bladder mastocytosis in a woman with chronic urticaria. Scand J Urol Nephrol 1997;31(5): 497-500.

(#28) Nerve and muscle disease (see also #76 below)

1. Lebbe C, Rybojad M, Klein F, et al. Schnizler's syndrome associated with sensorimotor neuropathy. J Am Acad Dermatol 1994; 30:316-318.

2. Lee HJ, Ahn WK, Chae KS, et al. Localized chronic urticaria at the site of Herpes Zoster. Acta Derm Venereol 1999; 79(2):168.

3. Kao NL, Zeitz HJ. Urticarial skin lesions and polymyositis due to lymphocytic vasculitis. West J Med 1995; 162(2):156-8.

4. Trueb RM, Pericin M, Winzeler B, et al. Eosinophilic myositis/perimyositis: frequency and spectrum of cutaneous manifestation. J Am Acad Dermatol 1997;37: 385-391.

(#29) Induction of urticaria by rubbing or scratching

1. Bruno G, Andreozzi P, Magrini L, et al. Mast cell activation in chronic urticaria-angioedema. Sci Total Environ 2001; 10 (270): 77-81.

2. Lin RY, Schwartz LB, Curry A, et al. Histamine and tryptase levels in patients with acute allergic reactions: an emergency department-based study. J Allergy Clin Immunol 2000; 106: 65-71.

3. Schwartz LB, Sakai K, Bradford TR, et al. The alpha form of human tryptase is the predominant type present in blood at baseline in normal subjects and is elevated in those with systemic mastocytosis. J Clin Invest 1995; 96: 2702-2710.

(#30) Painful swelling from sustained pressure

1. Barlow RJ, Warburton F, Watson K, et al. Diagnosis and incidence of delayed pressure urticaria in patients with chronic urticaria. J Am Acad Dermatol 1993; 29: 954-958.
2. Lawlor F, Black AK, Ward AM. Delayed pressure urticaria, objective evaluation of a variable disease using a dermographometer and assessment of treatment with colchicines. Br J Dermatol 1989;120:403-408.
3. Nettis E, Pannofino A, Cavallo et al. Efficacy of montelukast (Singulari®) in combination with loratadine (Claratin®) in the treatment of delayed pressure urticaria. J Allergy Clin Immunol 2003; 112(1):211-213.

(#32) Cold

1. Hoffman HM, Mueller JL, Brodie DH, Wanderer AA, et al. Mutation of a new gene encoding a putative pyrin-like protein causes cold autoinflammatory syndrome and Muckle-Wells syndrome. Nature Genetics 2001;29:301-5.
2. Hoffman HM, Wright FA, Broide DH, Wanderer AA, et al. Identification of a Locus on Chromosome 1q44 for Familial Cold Urticaria. Am J. Hum. Genet. 2000; 66:1693-8.
3. Rossa D, Tavoni A, Baldini C. Treatment of chronic hepatitis C infection with cryoglobulinemia. Curr Opin Rheumatol 2002; 14: 231-237.
4. Yu RC, Evans B, Cream JJ. Cold urticaria, raised IgE and HIV infection. J R Soc Med 1995; 88:294P-295P.
5. Wanderer AA. The spectrum of cold urticaria. Immunol Allergy Clin N Am 1995; 15: 701-723.

(#33) Exercise

1. Perkins DN, Keith PK. Food and exercise-induced anaphylaxis: importance of history in diagnosis. Ann Allergy Asthma Immunol 2002; 89:15-23.

(#35) Aquagenic urticaria

1. Parker RK, Crowe MJ, Guin JD. Aquagenic urticaria. Cutis 1992; 50(4):283-4.
2. Parks A, Camisa C: Aquagenic urticaria. Cutis 1986; 37(6):465-6.

(#36) Vibratory angioedema

1. Metzger WJ, Kaplan AP, Beaven MA, et al. Hereditary vibratory angioedema: confirmation of histamine release in a type of physical hypersensitivity. J Allergy Clin Immunol 1976 Jun; 57(6):605-608.

(#36A) Familial dermographism

1. Jedele KB, Michels VV. Familial dermographism. J Allergy Clin Immunol 1977;59:294-297.
2. Salazar Villa RM, Acosta Ortiz R, Mejia Ortiz J, et al. Symptomatic dermatographism and HLA antigens. Rev Alerg; 39: 89-95.

(#36B) Familial exercise-induced anaphylaxis

1. Grant JA, Farnam J, Lord RA: Familial exercise-induced anaphylaxis. Ann Allergy 1985;54:35-38.
2. Longley S, Panush RS: Familial exercise-induced anaphylaxis. Ann Allergy 1987;58:257-259.

(#38A) Familial aquagenic urticaria

1. Treudler R, Tebbe B, Steinhoff M, et al. Familial aquagenic urticaria associated with familial lactose intolerance. J Am Acad Dermatol 2002;47:611-613.

(#39) Hereditary angioedema

1. Bissler JJ, Aulak KS, Donaldson VH, et al. Molecular defects in hereditary angioneurotic edema. Proc Assoc Am Physicians 1997;109(2):164-73.

(#40) Muckle-Wells syndrome

1. Hawkins PN, Lachmann HJ. Interleukin-1 receptor antagonist in the Muckle-Wells syndrome. N Eng J Med 2003; 348:2583-2584.

(#44,#45). Animal exposure

1. Ewbank PA, Murray J, Sanders K et al. A double –blind, placebo-controlled immunotherapy dose-response study with standardized cat extract. J Allergy Clin Immunol 2003;111:156-61.

(#46) Arts and craft materials

1. DeGroot AC. Patch testing: test concentrations and vehicles for 3700 chemicals (2nd ed). Amsterdam, NY:Elsevier, 1994.

(#50) Medication history

1. Agostoni A, Cicardi M, Cugno M, et al. Angioedema due to angiotensin-converting enzyme inhibitors. Immunopharmacology 1999;44(1-2):21-25.
2. Barbaud A, Trechot P, Reichert-Penetrat, et al. Allergic mechanisms and urticaria/angioedema after hepatitis immunization. Br J Dermatol 1998; 139:925-926.
3. DeGroot AC. Patch testing: test concentrations and vehicles for 3700 chemicals (2nd ed). Amsterdam, NY: Elsevier, 1994.

4. Georgitis JW, Fasano MB. Allergenic components of vaccines and avoidance of vaccination-related adverse events. Curr Allergy Rep 2001; 1:11-17.

5. Grabbe J. Contact Urticaria. In: Henz BM, Zuberbier T, Grabbe J, Monroe E, eds., Urticaria 1998; 97-111, Berlin Heidelberg New York: Springer-Verlag, 1998.

6. Kaplan AP, Joseph K, Silverberg M. Pathways for bradykinin formation and inflammatory disease. J Allergy Clin Immunol 2002;109(2):195-209.

7. Karim M, Masood A. Fresh frozen plasma as a treatment for life-threatening ACE-inhibitor angioedema. J Allergy Clin Immunol 2002; 109:370-1.

8. Kleiner GI, Giclas P, Stadtmauer G, et al. Unmasking of acquired autoimmune C1-inhibitor deficiency by an angiotensin-converting enzyme. Ann Allergy Asthma Immunol 2002; 86(4):461-464.

9. Molinaro G, Cugno M, Perez M, et al. Angiotensin-converting enzyme inhibitor-associated angioedema is characterized by a slower degradation of desargininine(9)-bradykinin. J Pharmacol Exp Ther 2002; 303(1):232-237.

10. Oliver F, Amon EU, Breathnach A, et al. Contact urticaria due to the common stinging nettle (Urtica dioica)-histological, ultrastructural and pharmacological studies. Clin Exp Dermatol 1991;16(1):1-7.

11. Pasche-Koo F, Claeys M, Hauser C. Contact urticaria with systemic symptoms caused by bovine collagen in a hair conditioner. Am J Contact Dermatol 1996; 7(1):56-57.

12. Sanchez BM, Capriles-Hulett A, Cabello-Fonseca F, et al. Tolerability to new COX-2 inhibitors in NSAID-sensitive patients with cutaneous reactions. Ann Allergy Asthma Immunol 2001; 87(3):201-201.

13. Stevenson DD, Simon RA. Lack of cross-reactivity between rofecoxib and aspirin in aspirin-sensitive patients with asthma. J Allergy Clin Immunol 2001;108:47-51.

14. Sullivan TJ. Management of patients allergic to antimicrobial drugs. Allergy Proc 1991;12(6):361-364.

15. Uter W, Nohle M, Randerath B, et al. Occupational contact urticaria and late phase bronchial asthma caused by compositae pollen in a florist. Am J Contact Dermatol 2001;12:197-202.

(#52) Food history

1. Bernstein II, Storms WW. Practice parameters for allergy diagnostic testing. Joint Task Force on Practice Parameters for the Diagnosis and Treatment of Asthma.The American Academy of Allergy, Asthma and Immunology and the American College of Allergy, Asthma and Immunology. Ann Allergy Asthma Immunol. 1995; 75(6 Pt 2):543-625.

2. Goodman DL, McDonnell JT, Nelson HS, et al. Chronic urticaria exacerbated by the antioxidant food preservatives, butylated hydroxyanisole (BHA) and butylated hydroxytoluene (BHT). J Allergy Clin Immunol 1990; 86:570-575.

3. Hallett R, Haapanen LAD, Teuber SS: Food allergies and kissing. N Eng J Med 2002; 346(23):1833.

4. Henz BM, Zuberbier T. Most chronic urticaria is food dependent and not idiopathic. Exp Dermatol 1998; 4:139-142.

5. Keitel D, Amrol D, Marney S. Reduction of chronic urticaria with food dye and formaldehyde avoidance. ACAAI 2002 Meeting, Abstracts: Poster Sessions: 2002; P111, 48.

6. Lack G, Fox D, Northstone K et al. Factors associated with the development of peanut allergy in childhood. N Eng J Med 2003; 348:977-993.

7. Sampson HA. Peanut allergy. N Eng J Med 2002;346(17):1294-1298

8. Vadus P, Perelman B. Activated charcoal forms non-IgE binding complexes with peanut proteins. J Allergy Clin Immunol 2003; 112(1):175-179.

9. Venkatachalam M, Teuber SS, Roux KH, et al. Effects of roasting, blanching, autoclaving, and microwave heating on antigenicity of almond proteins. J Agric Food Chem 2002;50:3544-3548.

10. Vierk K, Falci K, Wolyniak C, et al. Recalls of foods containing undeclared allergens reported to the US FDA, fiscal year 1999. J Allergy Clin Immunol 2002;109(6): 1022-1029.

11. Zuberbier T, Chantraine-Hess S, Hartmann K, et al. Pseudoallergen-free diet in the treatment of chronic urticaria. Acta Derm Venereol (Stockh) 1995; 75:484-487.

(#54,#55) Disorders of the thyroid gland

1. Kandell AA, Zeid M, Helm T, et al. Evaluation of chronic urticaria in patients with Hashimoto's thyroiditis. J Clin Immunol 2001;21(5):335-447.

2. Leznoff A, Josse RG, Denburg J, et al. Association of chronic urticaria and angioedema with thyroid autoimmunity. Arch Dermatol 1983;119:636-640.

3. Rumbyrt JS, Katz JL, Schocket AL. Resolution of chronic urticaria in patients with thyroid autoimmunity. J Allergy Clin Immunol 1995;96:901-905.

(#56) Hyperparathyroidism

1. Armstrong JL. Chronic idiopathic (?) urticaria: a satisfactory outcome. Ann Allergy Asthma Immunol 1999;83:95-98.

2. Dagher HN, Aboujaoude ZC, Jabbour SA. Chronic urticaria: an unusual initial manifestation of primary hyperparathyroidism. Endoc Pract 2002;8:47-49.

3. Liechty RD, Firminger HI. Hyperparathyroidism and urticaria. JAMA 1983;250:789-790.

(#57A) Menstrual cycle

1. Lee CW, Yoon KB, Ju Yi, et al. Autoimmune progesterone dermatitis. J Dermatol 1992;19(10):629-631.

2. Mittman RJ, Bernstein DI, Steinberg DR, et al. Progesterone-responsive urticaria and eosinophilia. J Allergy Clin Immunol 1989;84(3):304-10.

3. Sharar E, Bergman R, Pollack S. Autoimmune progesterone dermatitis: effective prophylactic treatment with danazol. Int J Dermatol 1997;36(9):708-711.

4. Simpson G, Roomes D, Humphrey M. Anaphylactoid reactions associated with menstruation affecting two sisters. MJA 2001;175:415-417.

5. Slater JE, Raphael G, Cutler GB, et al. Recurrent anaphylaxis in menstruating women: treatment with a luteinizing hormone-releasing hormone agonist- a preliminary report. Obstetrics and Gynecology 1987;70(4):542-546.

6. Snyder JL, Krishnaswamy G. Autoimmune progesterone dermatitis and its manifestations as anaphylaxis: a case report and literature review. Ann Allergy Asthma Immunol 2003; 90: 469-477.

7. Yee KC, Cunliffe WJ. Progesterone-induced urticaria: response to buserlin. Br J Dermatol 1994;30(1):121-123.

(#57B) Hereditary estrogen-dependent angioedema

1. Binkley KE, Davis A. Clinical, biochemical, and genetic characterization of a novel estrogen-dependent inherited form of angioedema. J Allergy Clin Immunol 2000; 106(3):546-550.

2. Bork K, Barnstedt SE, Boch P, et al. Hereditary angioedema with normal C1-inhibitor activity in women. Lancet North Am Ed 2000; 356:213-217.

(#57C) Pruritic urticarial papules and plaques of pregnancy

1. Aronson IK, Bond S, Fiedler VC, et al. Pruritic urticarial papules and plaques of pregnancy: clinical and immunopathologic observations in 57 patients. J Am Acad Dermatol 1998;39:933-939.

(#58) Infections

1. Boyle JA. Mast cells: Beyond IgE. J Allergy Clin Immunol 2003;111:24-30.

2. Ostrov MR. Dramatic resolution of chronic urticaria. Ann Allergy Asthma Immunol 1995;75:227-231.

(#58B) Recurring infections of any type

1. Altschul A, Cunningham-Rundles, C. Chronic urticaria and angioedema as the first presentation of common variable immunodeficiency. J Allergy Clin Immunol 2002; 110(4):664-665.

2. Ballow M. Primary immunodeficiency disorders: antibody deficiency. J Allergy Clin Immunol 2002;109(4):581-91.

3. Busse PJ, Razvi S, Cunningham-Rundles C. Efficacy of intravenous immunoglobulin in the prevention of pneumonia in patients with common variable immunodeficiency. J Allergy Clin Immunol 2002;109(6):1001-4.

4. Cunningham-Rundles C, Bodian C. Common variable immunodeficiency: clinical and immunological features of 248 patients. J Clin Immunol 1999;92:34-48.

(#59) Jaundice

1. Daoud MS, Gibson LE, Daoud S, et al. Chronic hepatitis C and skin diseases: a review. Mayo Clin Proc 1995;70(6):559-564.
2. Kohler PF. Clinical immune complex disease. Manifestations in systemic lupus erythematosus and hepatitis B virus infection. Medicine (Baltimore) 1973; 52(5):419-29.

(#63) Wound infection

1. Edward A, Nolph K. Streptoccocal peritonitis with urticaria. Perit Dial Int 1992; 12(2):214-215.
2. Ostrov MR. Dramatic resolution of chronic urticaria. Ann Allergy Asthma Immunol 1995;75:227-231.

(#64) Infection of the sinuses

1. Altschul A, Cunningham-Rundles, C. Chronic urticaria and angioedema as the first presentation of common variable immunodeficiency. J Allergy Clin Immunol 2002; 110(4):664-665.
2. Cunningham-Rundles C, Bodian C. Common variable immunodeficiency: clinical and immunological features of 248 patients. J Clin Immunol 1999;92:34-48.
3. Liutu M, Kalimo K, Uksila J: Etiologic aspects of chronic urticaria. Int J Dermatol 1998;37(7):515-519.
4. Watson RD, Gershwin ME. Acquired angioedema associated with sinusitis. J Investig Allergol Clin Immunol 2000;3:129-134.

(#68) Fungal infections, i.e. athlete's feet, etc.

1. Platts-Mill TA, Fiocco GP, Hayden ML, et al. Serum IgE antibodies to *Trichophyton* in patients with urticaria, asthma and rhinitis: development of a radioallergosorbent test. J Allergy Clin Immunol 1987;79(1):40-45.

(#69) Skin infections and abscesses

1. Kravitz P, Stahl NI. Urticarial vaculitis, immune complex disease, and an infected ventriculoatrial shunt. Cutis 1985; 36(2):135-136,141.
2. Ostrov MR. Dramatic resolution of chronic urticaria. Ann Allergy Asthma Immunol 1995;75:227-231.

(#73) Sexually transmitted diseases

1. Lin RY, Schwartz RA. Cold urticaria and HIV infection. Br J Dermatol 1993;129(4): 465-466.

2. Purello-D'Ambrosio F, Gangemi S, Ricciardi L. Urticaria from *Trichomonas vaginalis* infection. J Investig Allergol Clin Immunol 1999;9(2):123-125.

3. Supanaranond W, Desakorn V, Sitakalin C, et al. Cutaneous manifestations in HIV positive patients. Southeast Asian J Trop Public Health 2001;32:171-176.

(#76) History of tumors, cancers

1. Alonso R, Cistero-Bahima A, Enrique E, et al. Chronic urticaria associated with chronic myelomonocytic leukemia. J Invest Allergol Clin Immunol 2000;10(6):380-381.

2. Clore LS, Stafford CT. Chronic urticaria as a presenting sign of hairy cell leukemia. Allergy Asthma Proc 1999;20(1):51-55.

3. Fremeaux-Bacchi V, Guinnepain MT, Cacoub P, et al. Prevalence of monoclonal gammopathy in patients presenting with acquired angioedema type 2. Am J Med 2002;113(3):249-251.

4. Govindaraju S, Brochet P, Ringot AC, et al. Chronic urticaria-macroglobulinemia (Schnitzler's syndrome): developing to IgM myeloma. Apropos of a case. Rev Med Intern 1993;14(8):780-783.

5. Greiner D, Schofer H, Boehncke WH. Urticaria associated with a small cell carcinoma of the lung. Cutis, 2002; 69(1):49-59.

6. Hills EA: Adenocarcinoma of the bronchus with Cushing's syndrome, carcinoid syndrome, neuromyopathy and urticaria. Br J Dis Chest 1968;62(2):88-92.

7. Kaplan M. Acquired C_1 esterase inhibitor with late presentation of lymphoma. J Allergy Clin Immunol 2002;109:S130.

8. Lewis JE. Urticarial vasculitis occurring in association with visceral malignancy. Acta Derm Venereol 1990;70(4):345-347.

9. Lipsker D, Cribier B, Maloisel F. Chronic urticaria and IgA myeloma. Acta Derm Venereol 1998;79(5):395.

10. Moward CM, Mowad JJ, Cirigliano MD. Testicular cancer presenting as urticaria. Cutis 1998; 61(3):147-148.

11. O'Donnell BF, Foulds IS. Thyroid carcinoma presenting as angioedema. Br J Dermatol 1993;128(5):588-589.

12. Razon S, Vegni M, Schiaffino E, et al. Ganglioneuroblastoma and urticaria by physical agents. Tumori 1990;76(3):282-285.

13. Reinhold U, Bruske T, Schupp G: Paraneoplastic urticaria in a patient with ovarian carcinoma. J Am Acad Dermatol 1996;35(6):988-989.

14. Shahar A, Sharon R, Lorber M, et al. Angioedema caused by splenectomy with malignant lymphoma followed by multiple myeloma 7 years later. Harefuah 1997; 132(9):624-626.

#77 through #83. History of environmental exposure through direct skin contact

1. DeGroot AC. Patch testing: test concentrations and vehicles for 3700 chemicals (2nd ed). Amsterdam, NY: Elsevier, 1994.

(#84 through #91A) History of autoimmune disease

1. Confino-Cohen R, Aharoni D, Goldberg A, et al. Evidence for aberrant regulation of the p21 Ras pathway in PBMCs of patients with chronic idiopathic urticaria. J Clin Allergy Immunol 2002;109:349-56.

2. Guillet G, Sanciaume C, Peyraud J. Inaugural skin manifestations of Still's disease: dermographic urticaria and pseudodermatomyositis. Sem Hop 1983; 59(24):1848-1851.

3. Mongia A, Wolff A, Bielory L. Mixed connective tissue disease with angioedema. Ann Allergy Asthma Immunol 2003; 90 (P113):147.

4. Payne CM, Thomas RH. Dermatomyositis with urticated lesions. JR Soc Med 1984; 77(2):137-138.

5. Ziegler A, Dinakar C. Systemic lupus erythematosus presenting as refractory angioedema in a 10 year old Caucasian girl mimicking drug allergy. (28) Ann Allergy Asthma Immunol 2003; 90 (#28): 103-4.

(#92) Anaphylaxis

1. Kemp S, Lockey RF. Anaphylaxis: a review of causes and mechanisms. J Allergy Clin Immunol 2002; 110(3):341-348.

2. Lin RY, Schwartz LB, Curry A, et al. Histamine and tryptase levels in patients with acute allergic reactions: an emergency department-based study. J Allergy Clin Immunol 2000;106:65-71.

3. Stark BJ, Sullivan TJ. Biphasic and protracted anaphylaxis. J Allergy Clin Immunol 1986;78(1,pt 1):76-83.

4. Tejador A. Idiopathic anaphylaxis. Ann Allergy Asthma Immunol 2002; 88:313-318.

(#93) Sexual intercourse

1. Didier EM, Perez T, Carre P. Anaphylactic manifestations during protected sexual intercourse disclosing allergy to latex. Rev Med Interne 1991;12(6):447-448.

2. Green RL, Green MA. Postcoital urticaria in a penicillin-sensitive patient. Possible seminal transfer of penicillin. JAMA 1985;254(4):531.

3. Greenberger PA. Allergy to sulfa drugs with postcoital urticaria. JAMA 1991; 265(11):1458.

4. Mike N, Bird G, Asquith P. A new manifestation of seminal fluid hypersensitivity. Q J Med 1990;75(276):371-376.

Treatment (Chapters 6 and 7)

1. Anand MK, Nelson HS, Dreskin SC. A possible role for **cyclooxygenase 2 inhibitors** in the treatment of chornic urticaria. J Allergy Clin Immunol 2003; 111:1133-1136.

2. Asero R. Are **IVIG** for chronic unremitting urticaria effective? Allergy Net 200; 55:1099-1101.

3. Bernstein JA, Garramone SM, Lower EG. Successful treatment of autoimmune chronic idiopathic urticaria with intravenous **cyclophosphamide**. Ann Allergy Asthma Immunol 2002;89:212-214.

4. Bork K, Barnstedt SE. Treatment of 193 episodes of laryngeal edema with **C1 esterase inhibitor concentrate** in patients with hereditary angioedema. Arch Intern Med 2001;161:714-718.

5. Botta RS, Grant JA, Jain VV, et al. Role of **montelukast** in chronic idiopathic urticaria. Ann Allergy Asthma Immunol 2002;88:114(P55).

6. Erbagci Z. The leukotriene receptor antagonist **montelukast** in the treatment of chronic idiopathic urticaria: a single blind, placebo-controlled, crossover clinical study. J Allergy Clin Immunol 2002;110(3):484-488.

7. Fadel R, Herpin-Richard N et al. Inhibitory effect of **ceterizine HCL** on eosinophil migration in vivo. Clin Allergy 17:373-379.

8. Finn AF, Kaplan AP, Fretwell R. A double blind placebo controlled trial of **fexofenadine HCl** in the treatment of chronic idiopathic urticaria. J Allergy Clin Immunol 1993;104(5):1071-1078.

9. Frossard N, Purohit A, Kovacs S, et al. **Fexofenadine** is superior to **loratadine** and **desloratadine** in onset of action of histamine-induced wheal and flare inhibition. Ann Allergy Asthma Immunol 2003;90 (#P34):124.

10. Gelfand EW, Cui Z, Takeda K. **Fexofenadine** modulates T-cell function, preventing allergen-induced airway inflammation and hyperresponsiveness. J Allergy Clin Immunol 2002;110(1):85-95.

11. Gach JE, Sabroe RA, Greaves MW, et al. **Methotrexate**-responsive chronic idiopathic urticaria: a report of two cases. Br J Dermatol 2001;145:340-343.

12. Grattan CE, O'Donnell BF, Francis DM, et al. Randomized double-blind study of **cyclosporine** in chronic idiopathic urticaria. Br J Med Dermatol 2000;143(2):365-372.

13. Greaves M. Management of urticaria. Hosp Med 2000;61(7):463-469.

14. Gupta MA, Gupta AK. Chronic idiopathic urticaria associated with panic disorder: a syndrome responsive to selective **serotonin reuptake inhibitor** antidepressants. Cutis 1995;56(1):53-53.

15. Hawkins PN, Lachmann HJ. Interleukin-1 receptor antagonist in the Muckle-Wells syndrome. N Eng J Med 2003; 348:2583-2584.

16. Jaffer AM, Tilden R, Erik R, et al. **Sulfasalazine** in the treatment of chronic urticaria. J Allergy Clin Immunol 2002;109(1):S127.

17. Kobza-Black A. Management of urticaria. Clin Exp Dermatol 2002;27(4):328-337.

18. Lawlor F, Black AK, Ward AM, et al. Delayed pressure urticaria, objective evaluation of a variable disease using a dermographometer and assessment of treatment with **colchicine**. Br J Dermatol 1989;120:403-408.

19. Lueng DYM, Sampson HA, Yunginger JW et al. Effect of **anti-IgE therapy** in patients with **peanut** allergy. N Eng J Med 2003; 348: 986-993.

20. Nelson HS, Reynolds R, Mason J. **Fexofenadine HCl** is safe and effective for treatment of chronic idiopathic urticaria. Ann Allergy Asthma Immunol 2000; 84(5): 517-522.

21. Purohit A, Duvernelle C, Melac M. Twenty four hours of activity of **cetirizine** and **fexofenadine** in the skin. Ann Allergy Asthma Immunol 2001;86:387-392.

22. Ring J, Hein R, Gauger A. Once-daily **desloratadine** improves the signs and symptoms of chronic idiopathic urticaria: a randomized, double-blind, placebo-controlled study. Int J Dermatol 2001;40(1):72-6.

23. Samuelson A, Towers TL, Ravetch JV. Anti-inflammatory activity of **IVIG** mediated through the inhibitory Fc receptor. Science 2001;291:484-486.

24. Shelley WB, Shelley ED: **Acyclovir** therapy for angioedema and chronic urticaria. Cutis 1997;59(4):185-188.

25. Simons KJ, Silver NA, Simons FER. Comparative study of H_1-blockade in skin produced by **fexofenadine, loratadine** and **chlorpheniramine**: correlation with plasma and skin concentrations. J Allergy Clin Immunol 2002;109(1):S161.

26. Simons FER, Silver NA, Gu X. Clinical pharmacology of H_1 **antihistamines** in the skin. J Allergy Clin Immunol 2002;110:777-783.

27. Stanaland BE. Treatment of patients with chronic idiopathic urticaria. Clin Rev Allergy Immunol 2002;23(2):233-241. (**tacrolimus**)

28. Tharp MD. Chronic urticaria: pathophysiology and treatment approaches. J Allergy Clin Immunol 1996;98(6 Pt 3):S 325-30.

29. Zuberbier T, Aberer W, Burtin B, et al. Efficacy of **ceterizine** in cholinergic urticaria. Acta Derm Venereol 1995;75:147-149.

30. Zuberbier T, Greaves M, Juhlin L. Management of urticaria: a consensus report. JID Symposium Proceedings 2001; 6(2): 128-131.

INDEX

ORDER FORM

Please send me _____ copies of **HIVES: THE ROAD TO DIAGNOSIS AND TREATMENT OF URTICARIA.**

U.S. **$29.95** per copy. Include **$6.00** for shipping and handling for up to 3 copies. Cost of S & H for more than 3 copies, and shipping outside the continental US will require an extra charge. Please contact AnsonPublishing LLC for a quote of extra charges.

PAYMENT OPTIONS

Check or Money Order payable to: AnsonPublishing, LLC

Circle Credit Card:

VISA   MASTERCARD

Card number _____

Expiration date _____

Name on card _____

Billing address _____

_____

_____

Phone _____

Shipping information (if different than billing address)

_____

_____

_____

Mail Order Form to:
AnsonPublishing, LLC
2055 North 22nd Ave., Suite 1
Bozeman, MT 59718
Telephone: 866-307-1112; FAX: 406-582-1112
E-mail: ansonpublishing@aacpc.com
For On-Line Orders:
www.alanwanderermd.com